Men'sHealth®

POWER TRAINING

BUILD BIGGER, STRONGER MUSCLES
THROUGH PERFORMANCE-BASED CONDITIONING

Robert dos Remedios, MA, CSCS
Foreword by Michael Boyle, MA, ATC

RODALE®

Men'sHealth

Printed in the United States of America
Rodale Inc. makes every effort to use acid-free ∞, recycled paper ♻

Book design by Anthony Serge
Interior photographs by Mitch Mandel / Rodale Images
Illustrations by Karen Kuchar

ISBN-13: 978–1–60529–885–6 hardcover
ISBN-10: 1–60529–885–9 hardcover

Distributed to the trade by Macmillan

2   4   6   8   10   9   7   5   3   1   hardcover

We inspire and enable people to improve their lives and the world around them
For more of our products visit rodalestore.com or call 800-848-4735

CONTENTS

4. THE POWER TRAINING WORKOUTS

5. POWER TRAINING EXTRAS

ACKNOWLEDGMENTS

This is a wonderful opportunity for me to recognize the many individuals who have helped and influenced me over the years. Thanks to Robin Pound, my college strength coach, for inspiring me to become a strength and conditioning coach. From you I learned that what we do is not only an art but a science as well. To my good friends and colleagues Jim Liston, CSCS, and Bill Hartman, CSCS. I have learned more from you folks than I could ever have learned in any book or class. To Michael Boyle, MA, ATC, who is one of the "originals" in this field and a great influence on my work. It's an honor to have you write the foreword. To Adam Campbell, thanks for introducing me to the world of fitness magazine writing—this is a big change from my everyday job! To my former assistant, Matt Durant, thanks for being a great worker and a great friend. I think I have learned as much as you during our thousands of discussions. To Mike Roussell, thanks for writing the nutrition chapter in this book; you *are* the next great nutrition expert in this field.

This list would not be complete without mentioning my good friend and colleague Alwyn Cosgrove, MSc, CSCS. You are one of the world's finest fitness experts for a reason. You are the real deal. Thanks for your help, support, and friendship over the years. I am excited about all the projects that lie ahead of us! And my assistant, Dustin Funk, CSCS. Thanks for all your hard work.

Thanks to the folks at Rodale Books for giving me this opportunity and taking a chance on a first-time writer. To my editor, Courtney Conroy, who inspired me to put my training philosophies and programs down on paper and get this book out to the masses. To Zach Schisgal for believing that a college strength and conditioning coach could actually pull off writing a book!

To my father, Abilio, who is responsible for the work ethic and determination that I have today. Without your guidance and examples, I would not be the man I am today. I miss you very much, Dad.

Lastly, to the two biggest loves in my life: my wife, Francine, and my daughter, Annabella. Francine, without your pre-editing of this book, the folks at Rodale would have been much busier. Annabella, you inspire me to be a better person. You two are the best. Thanks for all your support throughout this endeavor and through all the years.

FOREWORD

This is the type of book I wish I'd had when I was a kid. When I began to strength train in my teens, the only information available came from the muscle magazines that dominated our thought process in the 1970s. Oddly, in 2007, it seems as though we haven't come all that far. A visit to the gym today will find numerous trainees using outdated philosophies that stem from the bodybuilding days of the 1950s and '60s. But this book is a huge step in the right direction as we attempt to expose the public to the exercise concepts that have been used for more than a decade in the sports world. An old maxim says, "Learning always takes twice as long as it should. First you have to unlearn the old stuff, and then you have to learn the new stuff."

As a college strength and conditioning coach, Robert dos Remedios is bringing to the general public the information he's used to change the bodies and lives of thousands of athletes. The wonderful thing about books written by coaches is that they are written by those in the trenches. Robert dos Remedios knows that wins, losses, and college scholarships are at stake every time he trains an athlete. As a result, this program is designed to produce remarkable results for everyone who reads it. This is not a book written by a personal trainer or an armchair expert. This is a book written by a real guy who trains real people. In this age of the Internet, we are continually subjected to what I like to call "fake experts." These are the people who populate the chat rooms and the message boards that a lot of people visit to get (sometimes poor) exercise advice. It is easy to produce information, but it takes years of studying, practice, and experience to produce *good* information.

This book will help any competitive or recreational athlete, as well as those who just want to build a lean, strong, and powerful body to achieve their goals. The programs provided here are based on the latest research and are tested and retested in a real-life laboratory at the College of the Canyons in Southern California. This book is a product of real life and real training. A program developed by a coach who trains people every day for a living. Robert dos Remedios doesn't work with movie stars or talk-show hosts. He is not an expert because of the famous people he has trained. Robert is an expert because he trains hundreds of athletes *every single day*. No one knows better than Robert dos Remedios that training is about results, and this book will help you get them.

—Michael Boyle, MA, ATC,
Strength and conditioning specialist
and president of Elite Conditioning in Boston

INTRODUCTION

As a collegiate strength and conditioning coach, I work with hundreds of athletes every single day. Over the years, this amounts to thousands and thousands of "subjects" who have undergone my training programs.

In this book I've done my best to bring readers into the world of performance-based conditioning; a world where function comes first and physical benefits are unmatched. I see amazing physical transformations result from performance training, and I can honestly say that I have never used a single traditional bodybuilding movement pattern in any of our training programs. As I reflected back on the athletes that have come through and trained with me, I began to realize that their physical transformations did not happen by coincidence. The "athletic look" that most men want to achieve is developed by using very simple, effective training programs. At my level, I am given average athletes, and my job is to develop them into Division I level performers. Most of these individuals are just like you. My job is actually very different from the job of a strength coach who works with athletes already at professional or elite levels. If I fail in my task, my athletes will fail and their dreams of moving on are over. So, in no uncertain terms, my responsibility is profound. These bodies are being transformed at critical points in these athletes' lives, and I am in charge of this transformation. The programs I've developed over the years have helped hundreds of average athletes become Division I scholarship athletes and even NFL players. Because of the effectiveness of the programs, I believe the programs in this book can help anyone transform his body, get stronger and more powerful, and ultimately change his life.

Literally thousands of training programs are available to individuals who want to change their bodies. Most of these programs focus on the cosmetic aspects of body shaping, and therefore the typical body-part, muscle-building programs found in muscle magazines tend to dominate the industry. The problem with this is that these athletes, whose bodies and profound strength we seek to emulate, don't train using these traditional muscle-building training programs. These people train using performance-based conditioning methods like the ones in this book. By following these programs, these individuals develop well-proportioned bodies with few visible or functional weak-

IS TRAINING LIKE AN ATHLETE REALLY APPROPRIATE FOR *YOU*?

I think this statement from Nick Grantham, MSc, CSCS, who serves as regional lead strength and conditioning coach at the English Institute of Sport in Manchester, sums it up best: "For me, functional training means using the most appropriate training methods to enhance an athlete's performance. The key to success is selecting exercises that will maximize the transfer of training effect to ensure that what you do in the gym impacts directly on performance. If your training goal is to either improve your athletic performance or get into the best shape of your life, you cannot underestimate the value of functional training. I work with athletes from a wide range of sports. Not only are these athletes at the peak of their athletic ability, they have bodies that could grace the front cover of any health and fitness magazine. Believe me when I tell you that they don't get in that sort of shape by following traditional bodybuilding programs; it's purely a side effect of their no-nonsense, performance-based conditioning programs."

nesses or imbalances. In essence, these individuals are developing sought-after bodies and building tremendous strength without ever worrying about how jacked they *look*. These physiques, which we so badly want to attain, are, in fact, by-products of sound performance-oriented strength and conditioning programs—not old-school, single-muscle exercises or traditional bodybuilding programs.

Another big benefit of this training program is its *functional* nature. Whether you are a weekend warrior competing on the basketball court, a recreational golfer, or just a dad trying to keep up with his kids, this program will improve your performance. Your muscles will be stronger and more powerful, you will have great range of motion and flexibility, and most important, you will transform your body. Another aspect often ignored is that, at the end of the day, the integrity of our muscles, tendons, bones, and ligaments will all play roles in the quality of our lives down the road. In this respect, *everybody* is an athlete. This program will prove to be the best out there because it addresses all of these functional issues and at the same time it will develop strength, power, and athletic physiques.

Lack of time is the number-one reason people give for not adhering to training programs. Keep in mind that most competitive athletes have to balance training with practice, meetings, school, and so forth—not unlike most of our hectic schedules. Because of this, most athletic performance-based training programs are designed to be very time efficient without compromising results. This book goes a step further.

The training programs in this book are the most efficient and effective workouts on the market today. You will realize your physical potential through functional performance-based training—training methods used by some of the world's best-conditioned athletes. You will increase power, strength, and lean body mass using proven training techniques and an

"It's really simple: Train the parts that move your body in a way that makes them more efficient, and you'll get better results faster."

Adam Campbell, MS, CSCS,
Men's Health *magazine sports and nutrition editor*

unmatched menu of exercises. Regardless of your physical goals, the workouts to fit your specific needs are here. Getting in better shape, gaining muscle mass, or gaining strength—there is a workout for each of these goals. *Men's Health Power Training* contains the ultimate workout plan to help develop a chiseled athletic physique *and* gain strength and power in the most time-efficient and effective manner. The results will be unmatched by any other exercise program on the market today.

As an advisor to *Men's Health* magazine for several years, I have been able to share the exercises and programs I use with my athletes every single day and help incorporate them into the average *Men's Health* reader's training programs. Many of these exercises have never been seen before in any health and fitness magazine, yet they have always been received very positively. In fact, the feedback that I have received, at times, has been overwhelming. My experience in the normal gym setting has shown me that the general public is very curious about how athletes train and is looking for the most effective training methods available. This book will bring these one-of-a-kind training methods to the public for the first time and will change the way thousands of individuals will choose to train in the future. I guarantee that once you begin using these exercises, you won't go back to traditional training methods.

PART 1

UNDERSTANDING POWER TRAINING

WHAT ARE
STRENGTH AND POWER?

There are many ways to answer this question. Let's start by looking at the different types of strength out there. First, there's *muscular endurance*, which involves pushing, pulling, or pressing a load (weight) for multiple repetitions. Examples of muscular endurance would be performing as many chinups or pushups as you can possibly complete or choosing a submaximal load and performing as many reps as possible with this weight.

Next, there's *muscular strength*, which usually refers to pushing, pulling, or pressing a maximal load for 1 repetition. An example of muscular strength would be setting a world record in the bench press, which at present time is more than 1,000 pounds.

The last way to express muscle strength is through a static muscular contraction. An example of this would be a test of grip strength where you would squeeze a set of grippers and hold that grip for as long as you possibly can.

STRENGTH VERSUS SIZE GAINS

It's important to realize that approaching training for strength gains is a little different than training for size or hypertrophy (muscle growth) gains. While we can, and often do, observe improvements in both of these areas using one method of training, there are better ways to target each one.

SOME INTERESTING FEATS OF STRENGTH . . .

✔ Most pushups in 1 hour—3,416

✔ Most parallel dips in 1 hour—3,989

✔ Most chinups in 1 hour—445

✔ Heaviest power-lifting bench press—1,005 pounds

✔ Heaviest power-lifting squat—1,200 pounds

✔ Heaviest power-lifting deadlift—1,003 pounds

✔ Heaviest weight-lifting clean and jerk—580 pounds

✔ Heaviest weight-lifting snatch—469 pounds

If someone wants to improve his 1-repetition maximum (1RM) bench press or squat strength, he should be training with loads very close to maximum weight with fewer repetitions to gain maximal strength. On the other hand, if someone wants to get a larger chest or thigh muscles, he would want to train with higher volumes (sets + reps) and less weight to elicit a growth response.

In Chapter 4 , you'll learn how to determine which training goals and training cycles will help develop both of these variables. Remember this: *Any program that tells you that doing 10 sets of 3 repetitions will help you build size or that 4 sets of 10 repetitions will help you improve your 1RM on a particular lift is way off base, regardless of the prescribed load,* simply because these goals are dependent on both appropriate training volumes and loads.

THE ALL-IMPORTANT OVERLOAD PRINCIPLE

The most basic of all strength-training principles is the overload principle. Simply stated, this principle tells us that our bodies will adapt to whatever rigors we place on them. In other words, the more work you do, the more you will be capable of doing over time. With strength training, you can elicit an overload response by pushing harder during workouts. Increasing loads, increasing volumes, or even decreasing rest periods can accomplish this overload. There are no shortcuts here; the bottom line is that you need to push your body harder over time if you want to see improvements. The overload principle is not just spe-

cific to strength training; it can be applied to any physical training from flexibility to cardiovascular exercise. You'll see me stress this principle throughout this training program as it will be the key component to reaching your training goals.

THE LAWS OF SPECIFICITY

Much like the overload principle, the laws of specificity seem to state the obvious. If you want to improve your bench press strength, you need to bench press. In addition, you'll also need to consider variables such as loads, volumes, and frequency of training, since these things need to be specific to your training goals as well. For example, if I want to build bigger muscles yet all I do is 10 sets of 3 repetitions on all my exercises, I probably won't see the gains that I would want because hypertrophy is associated with higher volume sets than this. The example I like to use when explaining the laws of specificity is the 225-pound repetition bench press test used by the NFL and many other football testing combines. Oftentimes the person who gets the most repetitions is not the strongest bench presser as far as his 1RM goes. The strongest person is usually the one who has trained specifically for this test by doing multiple sets with submaximal loads to prepare his body for the endurance aspect. A person actually has to de-train his maximal bench press strength in order to improve his bench press *endurance* strength.

Despite the obvious nature of both the overload principle and the laws of specificity, it is not uncommon to see programs that claim to be effective yet ignore these very important factors.

MY BRAIN OR MY MUSCLES?

When a trainee starts a strength-training program for the first time, he usually sees results rather quickly. Typically, he might see increases in strength after only a few training sessions. Wow, did his muscles get stronger and bigger overnight? No. These initial improvements can be attributed to neural factors; that is, the body's central nervous system has figured out how to send the signal to the working muscles to be more efficient during the strength exercises. In other words, you always had that strength—you just didn't know how to use it.

After this learning or relearning process has taken place, improvements can be attributed to muscular or morphological factors such as muscle-fiber size increases or even anatomical changes in connective tissues. It is important to note that while initial strength gains may come in large amounts, the gains will eventually level off as the training continues. This is a normal progression for our bodies and one that should be considered when setting realistic training goals.

MUSCLE POWER OR MUSCLE STRENGTH?

While this book will emphasize both muscle strength and muscle power, the term *power* is often misused

POWER VERSUS STRENGTH

The simple equations to determine the strength and power in a specific exercise are as follows:

First let's look at a bench press performance . . .

Strength (work) = mass × distance

Example: 300-pound bench press that moves 2.5 feet

300 × 2.5 feet = 750 units of work

Power = work ÷ time

Example: The same bench press above takes 3 seconds to complete

750 work units ÷ 3 seconds = 250 units of power

Now let's compare this performance to a 100-pound power-clean performance . . .

Strength (work) = mass × distance

Example: 100-pound power clean that moves 5 feet

100 × 5 feet = 500 units of work

Power = work ÷ time

Example: The same power clean takes 1 second to complete

500 work units ÷ 1 second = 500 units of power

Note: Power exercises will always have higher amounts of power units than traditional strength exercises regardless of loads simply due to the time factor.

or misunderstood. The true meaning of power is the ability to generate as much force as fast as possible. A golf tee-off, a vertical jump, an Olympic clean and jerk, or swinging a softball bat are all examples of power. Basically, if you do these things slowly, they just won't work very well.

Strength, on the other hand, is the ability to generate as much force as possible with no concern for the factor of time. A 1RM bench press or a 1RM deadlift are examples of pure strength movements. It doesn't matter how long it takes to complete these tasks. All that matters is that it gets completed—doing it slowly doesn't take away from the success of the exercise.

Power, which is often referred to as speed-strength, is an important factor in sporting activities, but it is also used in everyday activities such as moving fast, running up a flight of stairs, or just keeping up with your kids. This book will incorporate power exercises into its program not only for these reasons, but also for the added benefits of these exercises such as increased caloric expenditure, increased work capacity, and increased overall body strength.

The power exercises that are listed and described in Chapter 8 are a part of each training session and will prove to be a vital ingredient in helping you to reach your fitness goals.

FUNCTIONAL TRAINING— REAL-LIFE STRENGTH!

HOW STRONG ARE YOU?

Ahh, the question heard around every gym on the planet. What are people usually asking about when they ask you how strong you are? Well, nine out of 10 times they want to know what you bench-press. How on earth did the bench press become the marker from which one is judged as strong or not strong? It's baffling when we observe the actual exercise and analyze its benefit in the real world. Don't get me wrong, as I think there are benefits to this exercise, but to label it as *the* exercise by which we judge strength is just plain silly. This chapter will explain why.

I will pose some questions to you. Who is stronger, the guy who can bench-press more than 400 pounds or the guy who can do 100 pushups nonstop? How about the guy who can squat well over 500 pounds versus the guy who can do 10 perfect, full single-leg pistol squats (page 76) with just his body weight? Okay, maybe that's not fair since one is a demonstration of maximal strength and the other is a display of muscular strength, endurance, and even balance. My point here is that there are many definitions of strength; some are just more applicable in the real world than others. There is only so much we can do with the strength that we develop from a bench press, but there are *lots* of things we can do with the strength we develop from an exercise like a standing push press (page 99).

The term *functional training* is not a new one. In fact, it is probably one of the most overused terms in training today. There is a phenomenon in fitness training where the pendulum tends to swing hard toward

> "What the experts call *functional training* is simply the application of common sense to weight training. Take what you know about science, throw out the old body-part junk, and it seems like what we have left over is what we now call functional training."
>
> *Michael Boyle, MA, ATC*

7

one end of a particular training trend spectrum. The case in point is this concept of functional training. There was a period when many trainers utilized what I like to call the "Cirque de Soleil" training method. The philosophy went that if we were not doing one-arm dumbbell shoulder presses while standing on one foot atop a BOSU Ball, then we weren't training for "real life" function. The problem with this philosophy is twofold. For one, how often do you find yourself having to press a weight overhead while standing on one foot on an unstable surface? The second problem is that the more instability we add to the equation, the less load we are able to handle. This type of training enables us to overload the central nervous system but rarely allows us to overload our muscular system. We know that an overload effect is necessary for size and strength gains. This is an example of a concept that might have had some merit but was taken to the extreme. The backlash to this philosophy was a hard swing of the pendulum in the other direction where trainers started to look upon this style of training (Swiss balls, balance boards, and so forth) in a very negative light. While many people tend to believe there is one superior way to train and that anything that doesn't fit within their training philosophy is worthless, I like to think that there is a place for many, many different types of training. Whatever works for my goals is what I want to be using.

The point I want to make is that when I talk about functional training, I am talking about just that—your ability to improve your everyday function via the *Men's Health* Power Training program. No nonsense,

no fluff, no gimmicks—just effective workouts. The movement patterns this program incorporates are movements we use every day. The exercises included in the program's menu are exercises that will get you bigger, stronger, and more powerful—and are influenced by many training philosophies.

Let's look at a few of these philosophical points—these points are adapted from Mike Burgener's *Power to the 4th* exercise guidelines.

1. **Train unsupported as much as possible.** This means that we should try to perform the majority of our resistance training while standing and not supporting ourselves with an outside object. Doing all of your training while supported (i.e., lying on a bench, sitting on a machine, and so forth) puts your body in a fairy-tale-like world in which core stability and balance are of no consequence. It has also been stated that you can only apply about one-third of your bench press strength when you attempt to use this strength while standing. Boy, that 300-pound bench press doesn't look very impressive anymore, huh?

2. **Train using primarily free weights.** Free weights, especially dumbbells, not only improve strength but also help promote muscle balance and increase range

> "Regarding Functional Training . . . are we still debating isolation versus integration?!"
>
> *Jim Liston, MEd, CSCS*

of motion simply by their unstable nature. They also go well with the unsupported points I just mentioned.

3. **Train "explosively" each workout.** I believe there are many benefits to explosive Olympic-style lifts. Even simple variations of the classic Olympic lifts such as the clean, snatch, and jerk can improve your overall strength and power, increase metabolism, and improve fitness not to mention benefits for balance, range of motion, and flexibility. In addition, there are tremendous strength benefits in trying to move loads as fast as possible regardless of the weight. It is this "intent" that is the key to fast-twitch muscle fiber development and therefore a huge role player in getting stronger and more powerful.

4. **Focus on compound exercises.** While I will talk more about multiple- versus single-joint exercises in this chapter, it is important for me to be up front about *Men's Health* Power Training philosophy on relying on multiple joint, compound lifts in its programs. Compound lifts are not only superior for building strength, but they are also more calorically challenging and elicit a greater endocrine response which results in elevations in testosterone and human growth hormone (HGH). In other words, you will get a boost to some great strength-building hormones each time we train with compound movements. These exercises are also much more functional than isolated exercises.

The other points of this training philosophy are the requirement that trainees push and pull in both vertical and horizontal planes, perform rotational movements, do knee- and hip-dominant exercises, and train *all* of these movements both bilaterally (two limbs) and unilaterally (one limb).

FULL-BODY VERSUS BODY-PART SPLIT ROUTINES

As I will continue to suggest throughout this book, body-part training is virtually a thing of the past. There is very little to be gained from training in isolated fashions. Not only is this type of training completely nonfunctional, isolated training might actually weaken muscle movement patterns in the real world. My colleague, Alwyn Cosgrove, once used a great example of this phenomenon when addressing the overuse of the leg extension exercise to isolate the quadriceps muscles. He said that not only are the quadriceps unable to function in this fashion (isolated knee extension) in everyday activity, the isolated training of this muscle group could actually be

> "Now before you ask me, 'Can I split up my routine in some way?' Of course you can. But split it up based on what your body *does*, not based on what 'part' it is. Splitting up by parts makes as much sense as splitting up by the number of freckles in that area."
>
> *Alwyn Cosgrove, MSc, CSCS*

weakening this muscle when we need to use it in a functional fashion, i.e., running or jumping, by confusing the muscle firing sequence since the quadriceps need to be activated in unison with the glutes and hamstrings to perform these tasks. The same would go for another overused isolation exercise, the biceps curl. Like the quadriceps, the biceps function along with the shoulder joint in everyday activity, *not* in isolated elbow flexion.

Are there some benefits to single-joint exercises? Sure. Bodybuilders rely on the aesthetic results of resistance training so isolation exercises can help increase muscle size in a targeted area. Keep in mind, however, that strength and functional ability is not a concern for most bodybuilders, so the issues I mentioned earlier generally don't mean much to them.

You will find that I have included a couple of single-joint exercises in my program. I do so only to address some common injury issues in the shoulder joint. These exercises are listed as replacement exercises in the vertical push menu category; the remaining exercises are all compound movements.

WHAT YOU CAN'T SEE *CAN* HURT YOU!

Another issue in training today is the tendency to train the "mirror muscles." This is a term I often hear Mike Boyle use when describing the way most people train in the gym. What he is referring to is the way many people only care about the muscles they can see when looking in the mirror. For example, people tend to focus on the shoulders, chest, abs, and even the

AN OBSERVATION AT THE GYM . . .

I belong to one of the bigger, more popular gyms in my area and decided one day to count how many people I would witness training the "unseen muscles" during my own training session. One thing I noticed for the very first time was the fact that there were *so* many more mirror-muscle machines and equipment compared to machines for the posterior muscle groups—a nearly 3-to-1 ratio! I also noted that not a single person (zero) trained hamstrings, lower back, or glutes (even in the form of a squat) the entire time I was in the gym. Keep in mind that I was there during a traditionally busy time of the day. These individuals are all depriving themselves of valuable muscle strength and balance, not to mention the potential for future postural problems and injury.

quadriceps while giving little attention to the upper and lower backs, glutes, and hamstrings. The muscles that we can't see in the mirror play a vital role in what is called our posterior chain. Neglecting these muscle groups not only leads to muscle imbalances—both in strength and appearance—but it also can lead to strength deficit issues that can result in injury. The Power Training program will always attempt to place equal emphasis on all muscle groups through its movement-oriented approach. Training volumes for all movements will be very similar at all times. In other words, if you push for 8 sets, you should pull for at least 8 sets as well. Besides, you don't want people to snicker behind you as they watch you walk away, right?

BILATERAL VERSUS UNILATERAL MOVEMENTS

First, some background on these terms. *Bilateral* exercises use both limbs in unison to move a load, such as barbell squats, barbell bench press, and chinups. If one limb pushes or pulls harder than the other, the load will not move evenly. *Unilateral* exercises focus on each limb working independently of each other. This can be accomplished by either isolating one limb at a time or by using dumbbells or independent stack cables to push or pull with both limbs at the same time. Examples of these movements include exercises such as dumbbell shoulder presses, dumbbell bent-over rows, and lunges. In addition, when unilateral exercises are performed one limb at a time, they can often elicit more core function due to the unbalanced state of the load. Examples of these types of unilateral exercises would be a one-arm dumbbell shoulder press or a one-arm dumbbell bent-over row. Unilateral work enables trainees to discover and address weaknesses and imbalances. This type of single-limb focus-

ing can also greatly improve bilateral movement strength. This can prove to be very effective if you are seeking improvement in exercises such as barbell squats, bench presses, and even pullups.

A unique aspect of the Power Training program is the inclusion of both bilateral and unilateral exercise options for almost all of the prescribed exercise movements.

All in all, the main goals of this book are to not only get you "stronger" in the traditional bench press, deadlift, or squat sense, but also to make sure that you are functionally sound as well. To me, strength is not just the ability to bench press or squat a large amount of weight. Being strong also means having the muscular endurance that enables you to do body-weight exercises like dips, chinups, pushups, or the balance and strength to complete a full one-leg pistol squat or hold a perfect core bridge for an extended period. This type of functional strength is very important for everyday activities and especially important for sport performance. By *my* definition of strength, the overweight guy who can bench-press 400 pounds yet not do a single chinup is not strong at all; he is a glaring example of what is wrong with many of today's training philosophies.

TOP 10 POWER TRAINING TIPS

Over the years, I've found myself changing my programs, exercises, and ideas fairly regularly. Sometimes things work well, other times they don't. There is a constant, ever-evolving educational process that comes along with working in the strength and conditioning field. My goal is to create the most effective, efficient training programs possible, so I regularly experiment with new ideas, exercises, and concepts that I either invent or borrow from other professionals. Here I have compiled a list of 10 tips I feel are extremely important in reaching your strength-training goals. These are tips I have incorporated for many, many years. In other words, while many other things come and go in my programs, these elements form the foundation of my training programs.

1. FULL FRONT SQUATS ARE VERY EFFECTIVE

Ahh, the almighty "king of the lower-body exercises." I can't say enough about this exercise. Full front squats may be the single best exercise on the planet. No other exercise imposes quite the demand that these place on your body. Let's take a look at some of the muscle requirements: wrist, shoulder, hip, knee, and ankle flexibility; core/torso, lower-back strength and stability; balance; and the obvious strength and power demands on the entire lower body.

Full front squats are an extremely taxing exercise that can expend a lot of energy and increase hormonal responses that can improve strength; these are very important benefits to anyone's strength-training program. The position of the weight makes the exercise more difficult than traditional back squats; therefore, you don't need as heavy of a load to elicit the same type of strength-gaining response from your body. Lastly, the placement of the bar also places less vertical stress on the spine, which is very important for your health and longevity.

2. OLYMPIC-STYLE LIFTS WORK THE ENTIRE BODY

This is where most people fail to get the most out of their strength-training programs. Many people are intimidated or are unfamiliar with Olympic weight-lifting exercises. To give you some background, these lifts include the clean and jerk and the snatch lift. While these are highly technical lifts that require an abundance of practice and proper coaching, there are many simple, highly effective variations of these lifts that still provide many of the same tremendous benefits.

The main purpose for which athletes use these Olympic-style lifts is for the rapid quadruple extension that occurs during what is called the second pull in any of these variations. This quadruple extension, as shown in the photo below, refers to the chainlike sequence of the ankles, knees, hips, and back forcefully extending to move a load as fast as possible. This rapid development of force results in extremely high power production levels.

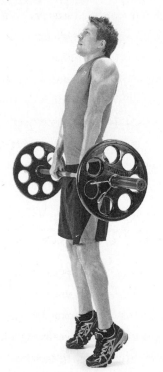

You are probably asking, "What does all this mean to the guy who is doesn't participate in any sports?" Well, these exercises are primarily total body exercises and require a lot of energy. This can result in greater fitness levels, increased caloric expenditure, and improved total body strength and power development, all of which can play a vital role in your training goals. Lastly, I personally like the improved balance, flexibility, and core stability that can result from performing these exercises.

Power exercises are obviously a big part of the *Men's Health* Power Training program and many Olympic-style lift variations from very basic to more advanced are included in this book. Keep in mind, however, that even the simplest movement, such as a clean pull (page 50), can be highly effective and elicit great power production, increase metabolism, and improve overall fitness.

3. DON'T FORGET SINGLE-LIMB EXERCISES

Squats, bench press, deadlifts, and even power cleans all involve using both limbs in unison. We also refer to this as bilateral training. The reality is that in most training programs, the majority of the exercises focus on these types of training patterns, which can often result in the dominant limb negotiating more of the workload than you'd think. There is a reason that a 400-pound bench presser will not be able to perform the same load when using two 200-pound dumbbells. First, each limb is now required to work independently

> "Total-body functional strength is the most glaring omission from almost all mainstream training programs today. This is especially true for the posterior chain, the muscles on the backside of your body. Poor development on the posterior chain not only leads to sub-optimal athletic performance, it creates muscle imbalances between the front and the back of the body—dramatically increasing the risk for injuries."
>
> *Adam Campbell, MS, CSCS,* Men's Health *magazine sports and nutrition editor*

4. HIP-DOMINANT EXERCISES FILL IN THE GAP

Most strength-training programs emphasize knee-dominant exercises such as squats, deadlifts, lunges, etc., and often exercises such as leg extensions and leg curls are added to "round out" lower-body training days. The problem with this type of program is its neglect of the very important hamstring and gluteal function of hip extension. In the bigger picture, incorporating hip-dominant exercises is the benefit of training the often-neglected entire lower posterior chain, which, in addition to the hamstrings and glutes, also includes the lower back. This book places much emphasis on hip-dominant exercises such as good mornings (page 82), Romanian deadlifts (page 85), and back extensions (page 86).

On another note, I recommend targeting the knee flexion function of the hamstrings and the calf muscles by performing exercises such as sled drags and hill or stadium walks rather than seated or lying leg curls (see Chapter 2).

5. IF YOU PUSH, YOU BETTER PULL AS WELL

Make sure you are dedicating as much time to pulling as you are to pushing in your training. Sounds quite simple, but analyze just about anyone's training program and you will most likely find there are significantly more pushing exercises than pulling exercises. By evening

(which will be foreign) and second, there is a higher level of instability that is not present when using a barbell.

By training unilaterally (one limb in isolation), we can detect and address existing weaknesses and imbalances. We can also improve our strength as we transfer this newly acquired strength back to the traditional bilateral exercises. This program promotes an equal amount of unilateral training in the form of exercises such as dumbbell push presses (page 102), several lunge variations (pages 68 to 71), one-arm lat pulldowns (page 113), and even single-leg good mornings (page 90).

out these two movements, we can assure better muscle balance in both size and strength as well as avoid the injuries that often accompany muscle imbalances between agonists (working muscles) and antagonists (muscles opposite of the working muscles).

In addition, you should make sure you are pushing and pulling in both horizontal (e.g., bench press [page 118], bent-over rows [page 134]) and vertical planes (e.g., push presses [page 99], chinups [page 108]). The shoulder-joint functions in all three planes and should be trained in all as well. Much like the overemphasis in pushing exercises, there is often a tendency to only push and pull on one plane.

> "If you look at the human muscular system—it's like a giant web of interrelated muscles. The lats run in a direct line into the glutes. The body was designed to function as a unit. Why we are sitting down and trying to separate this amazing machine and what it does into totally backward isolation exercises is beyond me."
>
> *Alwyn Cosgrove, MSc, CSCS*

6. DON'T SPEND MUCH TIME TRAINING YOUR CORE ON THE GROUND

The main purpose of your abdominals is to stabilize your torso. This stabilization occurs while standing, bending, twisting, lifting, etc., so it makes sense to spend more time training your core in these positions. Certain exercises like bridges (pages 165 to 167), which are very effective at building a stable core, are often performed on the ground, but not in the traditional "ab training" style of endless crunches and situps.

Also, training the core rotationally and on multiple planes will do wonders for your functional core strength and stability. Exercises using medicine balls not only build core strength and power but also improve range of motion and flexibility.

7. ISOLATED EXERCISES ARE OUT

As mentioned in Chapter 2, single-joint isolation exercises result in nonfunctional strength, confused muscle movement patterns, and possible weakening of "real life" muscle function. These things should throw up a big red flag when it comes to your training program. You will still target your biceps, triceps, quadriceps, and hamstrings using the compound exercises described here. The good part is that you will really be able to use all this new strength that you develop in the real world.

Remember that bodybuilders rely on isolation exercises for cosmetic purposes, not to get stronger. As far as building big muscles with isolation exercises, famous bodybuilder Milos Sarcev summed it up best when asked about whether bodybuilders are athletes. He stated, "We are not athletes, we are athletic mannequins."

8. CHANGE UP YOUR TRAINING WITH SOME STRONGMAN-STYLE EXERCISES

We've all seen those behemoths flipping 800-pound tires and pressing 300-pound logs, right? Sure, we may never get to that level, but we can come away with some great training ideas from their events. Most of these strongman events require total body effort, thus making them a very functional means of gaining strength and improving fitness levels. These types of activities also do a tremendous job of building work capacity, which can result in better efforts in the weight room. Try a few of the simple strongman exercises listed below and watch your overall strength and stamina improve by leaps and bounds!

• **Farmer's walk.** Grab a pair of heavy dumbbells and walk a set distance without putting them down. This is a killer on the grip, and increasing the load and distance will result in great overall body and core strength gains.

• **Car pushing/pulling.** Try pushing your car down the street. You can also buy a harness and pull it as well!

• **Tire flipping.** Go to a tire dealership that has large tires and see if you can take a used one off their hands. Squat down, get your hands under the tire, and drive it up to your hips then chest then over the top of your head.

• **Tug-of-war.** Not many activities can make your entire body work quite like a good old-fashioned tug-of-war!

• **Heavy sled dragging.** Get a strong piece of rope or other harness and tie a couple of heavy weight plates (or a car tire) to the end. Attach the other end onto a harness around your waist or shoulders (or just grab the rope) and pull away.

9. COMBINATION LIFTS CAN ADD VARIETY

Combination exercises involve combining two or more exercises In various patterns. Combining exercises gives you many benefits such as increased training volume, decreased training time, and more efficient space and equipment utilization. Combination lifts also allow us to unload or decrease our training intensity during long, hard training cycles. The interesting thing about combination lifts is that in addition to being a tool that can be used to decrease intensity, it can also be used to relatively *increase* training intensity when specifically used for this purpose. It tends to pack a lot of "bang for your buck" in terms of caloric expenditure and fat loss.

The Power Training barbell and dumbbell warmup sequence is, in fact, a combination lift called a *complex,* in which a series of exercises are completed back-to-back without resting. Lastly, throwing in combination lifts once in a while during a training cycle can be a great change-up and can help battle boredom and training plateaus.

10. PUSH THE ENVELOPE . . . IT'S OKAY!

There are all types of "quick fix" diets and "magical" exercise programs that promise us results with little to no hard work. Well, folks, I hate to burst your bubble but if you really want fitness results, it's going to cost you—in the form of hard work and sweat. If someone promises you results with a program that doesn't incorporate the basic principle of overload (see Chapter 4), they are lying to you.

The human body is maybe the most amazing creation ever. In addition to all the marvelous things that go on inside your body and brain, your body also shows great resiliency and actually thrives on overload. In addition, your body can take much more than the brain gives it credit for; acceptance of this fact is the biggest hurdle most people face. There is a comfort zone in which we feel most at ease and it is beyond this zone that we need to strive to train. It is at the point, when a repetition is brutally difficult or when that last set seems impossible, that we get the greatest results. It is when, because of this discomfort, you start to question why you are training or even why you are in the gym at all that you'll truly get the most out of your training. One of my favorite books is *The New Mental Toughness Training for Sport* by James E. Loehr, EdD. In this book, Dr. Loehr talks about a certain amount of discomfort that needs to be present in order to improve and that without this "personal confrontation," there can be little to no progress. Maybe it's the strength coach in me that comes out when I talk about this issue, but it is an issue I hold dearly. It's not only my athletes whom I demand this of; I demand it of myself every single day I go to the gym.

Now keep in mind that I am not telling you to go train blindly and ignore your body's signs and signals. Rather, I am telling you that overload and discomfort will and should be a part of your training. This discomfort is the reason most people out there don't train hard enough; it is also the reason most people never reach their fitness goals. Don't be afraid of it, thrive on it, and the results will speak for themselves.

PART 2
THE POWER TRAINING PROGRAM

PROGRAM DESIGN

When you're creating your training program, the first thing you need to complete is a needs analysis. In other words, you have to gather information regarding things like goals, training experience, available equipment, time constraints, and so on. Once you've completed this analysis, it'll be quite easy to incorporate *your* Power Training components and get started. Let's look at some of the things you will be asking yourself during your needs analysis.

GOALS

Depending on certain factors, your goals might vary when you start the *Men's Health* Power Training program. You might be interested in general fitness or getting in shape, or you may want to get bigger, or you may want to increase your strength and power for a particular sport. This program will facilitate virtually any training goal due to its unique and extensive menu of exercises and its periodization schedule. Let's look at some goal options:

• **Gaining size and/or changing shape.** These are common goals that focus primarily on the aesthetic results of training.

• **Increasing strength and power.** These are goals that focus on improving numbers on specific lifts and/or increasing power for sports performance.

• **Improving general fitness.** These are important goals that not only focus on getting stronger but also promote improvement of our overall health. This is more or less a "total package" style of training.

• **Meeting specific performance needs.** These goals are very specialized and can include things like improving your bench press max, increasing rotational core strength for golf, or even improving chinup endurance.

TRAINING EXPERIENCE

Much of how we train depends on our experience. Certain exercises are more difficult than others. In addition, how our bodies react and adapt to training programs depends on our experience. This program is not easy; *everyone* will experience discomfort, regardless of previous training experience. It is how you react to this soreness and discomfort that sets the tone for your entire training program. Remember, nothing comes easy and there are no magic tricks here.

If you are a beginner, the key will be to select appropriate menu exercises from each movement category and gain confidence and experience in these exercises. As your confidence builds, you will start choosing new exercises in each category. As training progresses, your body will adapt to the muscle breakdown and the effects of strenuous training sessions will gradually decrease.

For more advanced trainees, additional adaptation tends to be required due to the program's constant change of exercises and alternating linear periodization scheme. In other words, to continue to improve, the human body needs to work in cycles. By changing our exercises on a regular basis and by manipulating our volumes and intensities every few weeks, we will stimulate greater growth and strength. This will generally cause more soreness, even with advanced trainees, simply because of the workout-to-workout changes. Remember that change is a good thing and that the Power Training program incorporates this change to develop stronger, more functional bodies. For those advanced trainees seeking greater challenges, see Chapter 25 for additional training concepts.

EQUIPMENT AVAILABILITY

All too often our training programs are influenced, or even dictated, by the availability of certain pieces of equipment. I have created the Power Training program with this in mind. Almost every exercise listed in this program can be performed with a barbell and/or dumbbells. Although some cable exercise options are listed in the exercise menus, there are always barbell or dumbbell variations of these movements. Below you'll find a checklist of the essential equipment you'll need for the workouts in this book along with some inexpensive and important additions to your home gym.

Absolute Essential Equipment

- Olympic barbell and weights
- Dumbbells of varying weights or an adjustable set
- Adjustable bench or Swiss ball to use in place of a bench
- Fixed chinup bar (doorway style or tower)

Recommended Equipment

- Swiss ball
- Squat stands or power rack
- J.C. Band for rotational training and pulling (available at Perform Better, www.performbetter.com)
- Jump Stretch FlexBand for assistance on bodyweight exercises
- Medicine balls (3 to 5 kilograms)
- Weight belt to add weight to pullups or dips

Optional Equipment

- Dip bars
- Cable pulley tower

HOW MUCH TIME DO YOU HAVE TO TRAIN?

Time is the number-one factor in training adherence. Not many of us have unlimited time to spend in the gym, and I have made time an integral part of this program. The specifics of how this program will be implemented are found at the end of this chapter, but in general, you will be choosing from a 2-, 3-, or 4-day-per-week training schedule. Keep in mind that if you decide to follow the 2-day-per-week schedule, you will be spending more time in the weight room per session than if you had chosen the 3- or 4-day schedule, which requires less training time per session.

TRAINING CYCLES

First, some background on periodization. *Periodization* describes a plan of action in which loads and volumes are manipulated for specific training goals (i.e., hypertrophy, strength, power, etc.). There are generally two schools of thought in periodization. The first is *linear*, in which you train in a set fashion; you train for "x" weeks on hypertrophy, then "x" weeks for strength, then "x" weeks for peak strength and/or power, and then you repeat the entire thing.

A major training issue with traditional linear cycling is that, while you have a good amount of time to adapt to each training block goal, you can often end up being away from a particular training goal (for example hypertrophy), for many, many weeks, thus losing valuable gains.

The second school of thought is known as *undulating* periodization, in which you break up these training blocks every week, or even every workout, by constantly changing your sets, reps, and loads. For example, workout #1 in the week might address hypertrophy and workout #2 might target strength and so forth. One of the problems with an undulating cycling is that there is rarely enough time to adapt to any one mode of training, thus preventing maximum gains.

The Power Training program incorporates what I call *alternating linear periodization.* My close friend and colleague, Alwyn Cosgrove, coined this term, which means continually changing the volumes and loads during each training phase, but not to the extent of traditional undulating cycling. The program calls for changes in loads and volumes every 3 weeks. This ensures that you are adjusting to each training block *and* that you have enough time to adapt. Even more important, this method ensures improvement in your training based on the goals you've set for that training block. The other important aspect is that the trainee is never more than 3 weeks removed from either hypertrophy or strength training. The training programs detailed in Chapter 6 will give specifics, but a general example of alternating periodization would

SELF-ASSESSING THE HUMAN FACTOR

JIMMY—DAY 1

Jimmy goes to the gym to perform his Power Training workout. He stayed out a little late last night and didn't get much sleep. When he goes to do his normal weight of 100 pounds on the bench press it feels like a ton and he is unable to complete his reps.

What should he do?

Well, Jimmy needs to accommodate his physical state and understand that a workout's intensity is relative. In other words, on this particular day, his body will have to work just as hard to move, say 90 pounds, as it normally does to push 100 pounds. All that matters is the fact that he is still working to capacity and completing the workout. His brain knows that this is not 100 pounds, but his body couldn't care less.

JIMMY—DAY 2

Jimmy gets to the gym to do his workout and gets under the squat bar. He instantly notices that the weights seem much lighter today. He is normally able to do a set of 10 reps with 180 pounds, but today this load feels 20 to 30 pounds lighter than normal.

What should he do?

Okay, for whatever reason, Jimmy feels very strong today. It would be counterproductive to just go through the motions and do his usual sets and reps with a load that feels very easy. Therefore, he needs to add weight to his sets. My suggestion is to increase the load as much as he can while still remaining within the targeted set/rep scheme. You never know when or how often these "strong days" will come around so you must take advantage of them when they arrive! The opportunity to handle heavier loads is a big bonus to your strength-training goals.

be 3 weeks of higher-volume hypertrophy work, followed by 3 weeks of low-volume strength training, followed by 3 weeks of medium-volume hypertrophy training, etc.

TRAINING VOLUMES

Training volume refers to the amount of load, reps per set, and total sets per workout. For example, 4 sets of 10 repetitions on the bench press with 100 pounds would have a volume of 4,000 pounds ($4 \times 10 \times 100$).

Higher volumes and moderate loads (weight) during workouts characterize hypertrophy training, while lower volumes and higher loads characterize strength training. There are no two ways about these training volumes. To get bigger, you will need to handle moderate loads for numerous sets and repetitions, and to get stronger, you will need to handle heavy loads for fewer repetitions. There is nothing glamorous or sexy about this. In fact, there should be significant discomfort and fatigue as a result of hypertrophy training with these "moderate" loads—even more so than the lower-volume, higher-load strength training. In spite of the claims of the abundant fad-style training programs, this is just the reality of resistance training.

LOAD ASSIGNMENT

One of the great training questions of all time is, "How much weight should I use for each set?" Well, my response usually is, "What are you training for?" As I mentioned earlier, you will use relatively lighter loads if you are training for hypertrophy than if you are training for strength. If you're training for strength, use heavier loads. One thing that everyone needs to remember is the overload principle I mentioned earlier, which states that in order to improve our training, we must constantly train to elicit an overload effect. It isn't good enough to say that you completed a set of 10 reps with 100 pounds if you were actually able to do, say, 12 or more reps with that weight. Your goal should be to get the most work out of each and every set that you perform during these workouts.

THE HUMAN FACTOR

One pet peeve that I have with many training programs is when the program calls for a trainee to use say 60, 65, and then 70 percent of his 1-repetition maximum (1RM) when performing sets of 10 reps in sort of a "building up" fashion. My problem is that 70 percent of a 1RM tends to be about the average 10-repetition maximum load. So in doing a workout like this, we won't be reaching any point of overload until around our last set, thus wasting valuable time and effort. The other problem is that programs that prescribe specific loads for each set don't account for what I call the *human factor*. This factor is constantly changing based on fatigue, soreness, good days, bad days, etc. So while I will give you approximate training loads based on percentages of your 1RM, I realize there will be days when you will be weaker and days when you will be stronger. The key to building a solid training program is your ability to recognize and accommodate weaker days by lowering

loads at times, and taking advantage of those days when you feel stronger than ever by increasing the weights.

LOAD ESTIMATION CHARTS

On the next page of this book, you'll find estimated percentage charts based on your 1RM. These are prescribed loads that could be used for a certain amount of repetitions. There are a couple of drawbacks to these charts. The first is the fact that you would actually have to determine your 1RM on every single exercise you perform. The second is that it is impossible to assign an *exact* percentage, as these are merely estimates that will vary from person to person. I have included them as a reference so that you would have a means of predicting your 1RM based on your training sets. You can look at this chart from two viewpoints. First, you can determine your 1RM load and then calculate approximately what load you should be using. For example, if your 1RM is 130 pounds and you are doing sets of 10 reps, you would use a load close to 90 pounds (find your 1RM under the "max" column and now look across to the right to find the amount of reps you want to perform). The other way you can look at it is to estimate your 1RM based on a load used in your training sets. For example, suppose your best set of 5 reps on front squats is 100 pounds. It is safe to estimate that your 1RM would be around 120 pounds (find the 5 reps at the top and look down to find your best 5-rep load).

LOAD ESTIMATION BASED ON PERCENTAGES

REPS	15	12	10	8	6	5	4	3	2
MAX	60%	65%	70%	75%	82%	85%	87%	90%	92%
50	30	33	35	38	41	43	44	45	46
60	36	39	42	45	49	51	52	54	55
70	42	46	49	53	57	60	61	63	64
80	48	52	56	60	66	68	70	72	74
90	54	59	63	68	74	77	78	81	83
100	60	65	70	75	82	85	87	90	92
110	66	72	77	83	90	94	96	99	101
120	72	78	84	90	98	102	104	108	110
130	78	85	91	98	107	111	113	117	120
140	84	91	98	105	115	119	122	126	129
150	90	98	105	113	123	128	131	135	138
160	96	104	112	120	131	136	139	144	147
170	102	111	119	128	139	145	148	153	156
180	108	117	126	135	148	153	157	162	166
190	114	124	133	143	156	162	165	171	175
200	120	130	140	150	164	170	174	180	184
210	126	137	147	158	172	179	183	189	193
220	132	143	154	165	180	187	191	198	202
230	138	150	161	173	189	196	200	207	212
240	144	156	168	180	197	204	209	216	221
250	150	163	175	188	205	213	218	225	230
260	156	169	182	195	213	221	226	234	239
270	162	176	189	203	221	230	235	243	248
280	168	182	196	210	230	238	244	252	258
290	174	189	203	218	238	247	252	261	267
300	180	195	210	225	246	255	261	270	276
310	186	202	217	233	254	264	270	279	285
320	192	208	224	240	262	272	278	288	294
330	198	215	231	248	271	281	287	297	304
340	204	221	238	255	279	289	296	306	313
350	210	228	245	263	287	298	305	315	322
360	216	234	252	270	295	306	313	324	331
370	222	241	259	278	303	315	322	333	340
380	228	247	266	285	312	323	331	342	350

LOAD ESTIMATION BASED ON PERCENTAGES (*continued*)

REPS	15	12	10	8	6	5	4	3	2
MAX	60%	65%	70%	75%	82%	85%	87%	90%	92%
390	234	254	273	293	320	332	339	351	359
400	240	260	280	300	328	340	348	360	368
410	246	267	287	308	336	349	357	369	377
420	252	273	294	315	344	357	365	378	386
430	258	280	301	323	353	366	374	387	396
440	264	286	308	330	361	374	383	396	405
450	270	293	315	338	369	383	392	405	414
460	276	299	322	345	377	391	400	414	423
470	282	306	329	353	385	400	409	423	432
480	288	312	336	360	394	408	418	432	442
490	294	319	343	368	402	417	426	441	451
500	300	325	350	375	410	425	435	450	460
510	306	332	357	383	418	434	444	459	469
520	312	338	364	390	426	442	452	468	478
530	318	345	371	398	435	451	461	477	488
540	324	351	378	405	443	459	470	486	497
550	330	358	385	413	451	468	479	495	506
560	336	364	392	420	459	476	487	504	515
570	342	371	399	428	467	485	496	513	524
580	348	377	406	435	476	493	505	522	534
590	354	384	413	443	484	502	513	531	543
600	360	390	420	450	492	510	522	540	552

REST PERIODS

How long should you rest between sets? This again will depend on your training goals and the specific exercises you are performing. In general, it takes longer to recover from compound exercises than isolated exercises due to the amount of work being performed. Also, when training for strength, it is important to have adequate recovery time to be able to efficiently perform additional sets with these heavy loads. With the explosive exercises I have included in this program, it is important to recover nearly completely so that form will not be compromised. With hypertrophy, rest periods will be rather short to promote fatigue and to elicit maximal size gains. All the exercises here have predetermined rest periods based on this rationale (see the table below).

Another option I've included in these workouts is

REST PERIODS BETWEEN SETS

EXERCISES	2–5 REPS	4–6 REPS	8–10 REPS
Power exercises	2 min	n/a	n/a
All other exercises	90 sec–2 min	90 sec–2 min	60 sec

the option to *pair* exercises to cut down on training time. This technique allows you to move back and forth from one exercise to another to target a different muscle group(s) after each set and/or to speed up your training without compromising recovery time of the working muscles. Commonly called *super-setting*, this exercise pairing is a great way to kick-start your training sessions, but it usually requires the use of two pieces of equipment, which may be problematic in a commercial gym setting. Due to the pairing of "opposite" strength movements, these pairings are included in the full-body workouts, but not the push-pull workouts. The option to complex sets is described in the advanced training chapter (Chapter 24).

TRAINING TEMPO

Tempo refers to the amount of time it takes to perform both the concentric phase (the time it takes for the working muscle to shorten) and the eccentric or negative phase of an exercise (the time it takes for the working muscle to lengthen). Using the bench press as an example, the eccentric phase occurs when the weight is lowered to the chest and the concentric phase occurs as the weight is pressed upward to full extension. There have been numerous theories regarding the benefits of tempo manipulation and even extremely slow tempo techniques on training effectiveness. There has been little research to prove that this type of training is superior to traditional tempo training. While it makes sense that you would feel more fatigued and even have more soreness when training with very slow tempos (due to the extended eccentric phase), this should not be confused with training progress. The Power Training program utilizes what I call a *realistic training tempo*. Weight is lowered in a controlled fashion, and raised as fast as possible. With this in mind, I have estimated that it takes approximately 2 seconds to complete a repetition of any given exercise. Lastly, remember that "moving the weight as fast as possible" is a relative statement. When training with heavier loads, it will be impossible to actually move the weight fast. While you will try to move the weight as fast as possible, it will still appear to be move quite slowly at times. Keep in mind that this is an important aspect of training as the intent to move a weight as fast as possible is a key to improving strength and power during training.

WARMUP AND MOBILITY PROGRAM

The purpose of a pre-exercise session warmup is to prepare your body for the rigors that are about to be placed on it. There are various schools of thought on how to warm up, how long the warmup should last, and even if a warmup is necessary before lifting. While I have mentioned that time is a key factor in your workouts, I don't want to compromise the well-being of your muscles, tendons, and joints for the sake of saving time. I have put together a very sound warmup that can be completed in as short as 7 minutes, and I am confident that it will be very effective at readying your body for a training session.

The *Men's Health* Power Training warmup sequence is an efficient plan that will help warm up your body, improve range of motion by increasing the elasticity of your muscles and tendons, and prepare your body for specific exercise movements in a simple, three-step program. These three steps are:

1. Warmup
2. Mobility circuit
3. Specific lifting complex (see Chapter 17)

WARMUP

The purpose of the warmup is to increase your body temperature to help improve your muscle and tendon pliability in order to facilitate an improved range of motion. Trying to elongate your muscles when they are not warm is a futile and usually ineffective practice. I prescribe a 3- to 5-minute brisk aerobic-style warmup to increase body core temperature. This can come in the form of a light jog, jump rope, rowing machine, or even jogging in place or doing jumping jacks. Find something that you enjoy and just do it. While many programs advise a 5- to 10-minute aerobic-style warmup, I find that doing this for longer than 5 minutes tends to be a bit of overkill especially since the mobility circuit and specific lifting pattern warmup that I incorporate will keep your heart rate pretty high due to their dynamic properties. At the end of your 3- to 5-minute warmup, you will move directly into the mobility patterns described next.

29

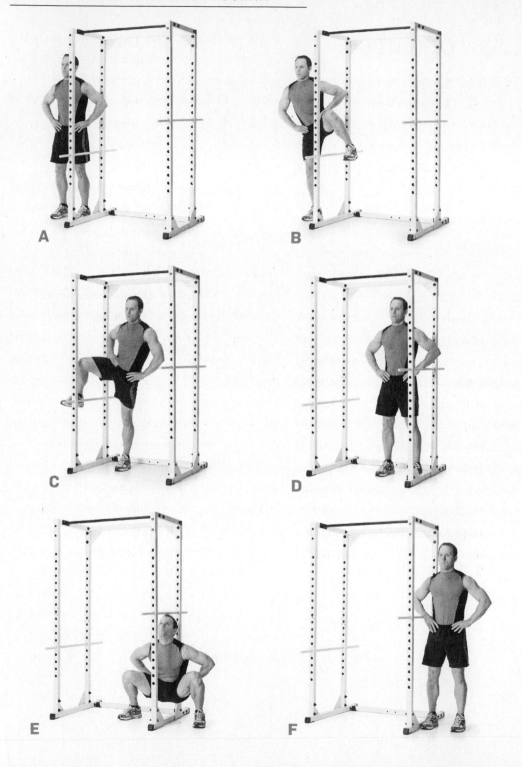

MOBILITY CIRCUIT

The mobility movements are considered to be dynamic flexibility patterns. This means they help improve range of motion by elongating muscles during an active movement pattern as opposed to a static stretching method. The patterns include the following movements:

1. Over/under hurdle—lateral
2. Over/under hurdle—forward

You can use the adjustable spotter bars of a standard squat rack to facilitate the hurdle patterns. If these are unavailable, simply use your imagination and step over and under imaginary hurdles during your movement patterns, making sure to step as high as possible and squat as low as possible as you move over and under both laterally and forward. You will have one bar set high (that you will move under) and one set lower (that you will move under).

Over/under hurdle—lateral. Standing perpendicular to the bars (A), keep your shoulders square as you move laterally, stepping over the first bar (B). Be sure to take a big step so you will be able to bring your back leg over the bar as you move to your right (C). Try to make sure that no part of your body touches the bar at all. As you move toward the next bar (D), step under the bar using a big step and drop as low as possible (E), trying not to bend over at the waist too much to get under the bar. Try to keep your eyes up as this will help maintain a tall torso and create greater range of motion in your ankles, knees, hips, and groin (F). Now make your way back through the hurdles moving to your left, beginning with the "under" phase and ending with the "over" phase. This is 1 repetition. You will complete 2 reps before progressing to the next movement.

Over/under hurdle—forward. Very similar to the lateral movement except that now you will face the bars. Using a big step, step over with your right leg and bring your trail leg up and over, trying not to touch any part of the bar. Attempt to keep your shoulders and hips square to the bar the whole time. As you come up to the next bar, take a big step under the bar with your right leg, drop your head slightly, and move under the bar without touching it. Turn around and come back through the hurdles, starting with your left leg stepping under first and finishing by stepping over with your left foot at the second bar. This is 1 repetition. You will complete 2 reps.

UNDERSTANDING THE POWER TRAINING WORKOUTS

Okay, so you know where I stand regarding isolated body-part training, so it won't be a surprise to find that there are virtually no single-joint exercises in the Power Training program.

Where you might have found an abundance of programs in the past that had a back + biceps day, a chest + triceps day, and even a quads + calves day, you will perform this program either as a full-body workout or a push-pull workout, depending on your preferences and based on your needs analysis.

Following are workout templates, exercise menus, training schedules, and estimated program durations.

THE POWER TRAINING WORKOUT TEMPLATES

Workouts are either split into a full-body sequence or a push-pull sequence, depending on the number of days you intend to train and how much time you have available per session. In addition, you will notice that for most movements, you will be assigned a bilateral exercise one day and a unilateral exercise for your next workout. In a nutshell, below are the movement templates for your workouts. Simply follow the template and pick and choose from the menu:

FULL BODY

WORKOUT A	WORKOUT B
1. Explosive Movement	1. Explosive Movement
2. Knee Dominant (bi)	2. Knee Dominant (uni)
3. Hip Dominant (uni)	3. Hip Dominant (bi)
4. Horizontal Push (bi)	4. Horizontal Push (uni)
5. Horizontal Pull (uni)	5. Horizontal Pull (bi)
6. Vertical Push (bi)	6. Vertical Push (uni)
7. Vertical Pull (uni)	7. Vertical Pull (bi)
8. Rotational/Bridge Core	8. Rotational/Bridge Core

Uni = unilateral, bi = bilateral

PUSH-PULL

WORKOUT A1 (PUSH)	WORKOUT B1 (PULL)
1. Explosive Movement	1. Explosive Movement
2. Knee Dominant (bi)	2. Hip Dominant (uni)
3. Horizontal Push (uni)	3. Horizontal Pull (bi)
4. Vertical Push (bi)	4. Vertical Pull (uni)
5. Rotational/Bridge Core	5. Rotational/Bridge Core
WORKOUT A2 (PUSH)	**WORKOUT B2 (PULL)**
1. Explosive Movement	1. Explosive Movement
2. Knee Dominant (uni)	2. Hip Dominant (bi)
3. Horizontal Push (bi)	3. Horizontal Pull (uni)
4. Vertical Push (uni)	4. Vertical Pull (bi)
5. Rotational/Bridge Core	5. Rotational/Bridge Core

Uni = unilateral, bi = bilateral

PERFORMING THE POWER TRAINING WORKOUTS

The unique characteristic and key component in this program is the large menu of exercises. This menu gives you a multitude of options so your training will never get stagnant. In fact, I encourage you to try to perform each and every exercise listed in the menu at some point in your training. This menu and the vast selection and variety of exercises listed for each movement pattern are what make this program different from anything currently on the market. Based on the training template you choose, you will select an exercise from each movement category in the menus below to perform each session. In other words, if the template calls for a bilateral horizontal pull movement, refer to that area of the menu and select the exercise of your choice.

Too often, we get stuck in a particular routine and almost get *too* comfortable in our exercise selection. Regularly changing up exercises not only fights boredom and plateaus but also improves muscle balance and strength. With the variety in this extensive menu, you are almost forced to try new exercises.

EXPLOSIVE EXERCISE MENU

Squat Jump
Hang Jump Shrug
Clean Pull
Snatch Pull
Clean High Pull
Snatch High Pull
Hang Power Clean (barbell and dumbbell)

Power Clean (barbell and dumbbell)
Hang Power Snatch (barbell and dumbbell)
Muscle Snatch
Power Snatch (barbell and dumbbell)
Narrow-Grip Power Snatch
One-Arm Dumbbell Snatch

KNEE-DOMINANT EXERCISE MENU

BILATERAL	UNILATERAL
Front Squat	Forward Lunge
Back Squat	Reverse Lunge
Overhead Squat	Side Lunge
Split Squat	Drop Lunge
Side Squat	Stepup
Clean-Grip Deadlift	Lateral Stepup
	Bulgarian Split Squat
	Bulgarian Split Deadlift
	Single-Leg Bench Getup
	Crouching Single-Leg Squat
	Partial Single-Leg Squat Using a Bench or Box for Depth
	Partial Single-Leg Squat Standing on a Bench
	Single-Leg Squat Standing on a Bench
	Single-Leg Squat (lateral)
	Full Pistol Squat

HIP-DOMINANT EXERCISE MENU

BILATERAL	UNILATERAL
Good Morning	Single-Leg Good Morning
Seated Good Morning	Split Good Morning
Zercher Good Morning	Single-Leg Romanian Deadlift
Romanian Deadlift	Single-Leg Romanian Deadlift (dumbbell)
Back Extension	Single-Leg Back Extension
Supine Hip Extension	Single-Leg Supine Hip Extension
Swiss Ball Glute-Hamstring	Single-Leg Swiss Ball Glute-Hamstring
Reverse Hyperextension	

VERTICAL PUSH EXERCISE MENU

BILATERAL	UNILATERAL
Shoulder Press	Dumbbell Shoulder Press
Push Press	Dumbbell Push Press
Push Jerk	Dumbbell Push Jerk
Split Jerk	Dumbbell Split Jerk
Jackknife Pushup	Dumbbell One-Arm Press + Bend
*Plate Raise + Truck Driver	Dumbbell Alternating Press
	Supported Dumbbell One-Arm Press
	Side-to-Side Jackknife Pushup
	*Dumbbell Parallel-Grip Push Press
	*Dumbbell Scaption
	*Dumbbell Scaption with Shrug

*See "Shoulder Considerations" in Chapter 11 for exercise instructions.

VERTICAL PULL EXERCISE MENU

BILATERAL	UNILATERAL
Chinup	Single-Arm Pullup
Pullup	Single-Arm Lat Pulldown
Mixed-Grip Pullup	Side-to-Side Pullup
Lat Pulldown	
*Parallel-Grip Pullup/Pulldown	

*This exercise is a variation for someone with a shoulder injury.

HORIZONTAL PUSH EXERCISE MENU

BILATERAL	UNILATERAL
Bench Press	Dumbbell Bench Press
Incline Bench Press	Dumbbell Incline Bench Press
Close-Grip Bench Press	Dumbbell Alternating Bench Press
Close-Grip Incline Press	One-Arm Dumbbell Bench Press
Reverse-Grip Bench Press	One-Arm Dumbbell Incline Bench Press
Pushup (floor, ball, chair)	Side-to-Side Pushup
Dip	Standing Cable Chest Press

HORIZONTAL PULL EXERCISE MENU

BILATERAL	UNILATERAL
Bent-Over Row	Bent-Over Dumbbell Alternating Row
Modified T-Bar Row	Bent-Over Two-Point Dumbbell Row
Horizontal Pullup	Two-Point Dumbbell Row with Twist
Standing Cable Row to Ribcage	One-Arm Standing Cable Row
Standing Cable Row to Neck	Horizontal Side-to-Side Pullup
*Cable Face Pull	One-Arm Horizontal Pullup

*See "Rehab Corner" in Chapter 14 for exercise instructions.

ROTATIONAL CORE EXERCISE MENU

Seated Russian Twist	Cable Wood Chop
Corkscrew	Cable Rotating Crunch
Swiss Ball Weight Roll	Cable Rotating Extension
Barbell Torque	Cable Push-Pull Rotation
Windshield Wiper	Medicine Ball Standing Wall Throw
Cable Rotation	Medicine Ball Over-the-Shoulder Throw and Catch
Cable Reverse Wood Chop	Medicine Ball 1-2-3 Throw

BRIDGING AND CORE STABILIZATION EXERCISE MENU

Four-Point Plank	Plank with Elbow to Knee
Three-Point Plank	Plank Walkup
Two-Point Plank	Plank with Weight Transfer
Side Bridge	Side Bridge and Reach
Four-Point Supine Bridge	Core Row
Three-Point Supine Bridge	T-Push and Hold
Dynamic Plank	Barbell Rollout

WARMUP COMPLEXES

BARBELL COMPLEX
1. Hang Power Shrug
2. Hang Power Clean
3. Push Press
4. Front Squat
5. Bent-Over Row
6. Romanian Deadlift

WARMUP COMPLEXES (*cont.*)

DUMBBELL COMPLEX
1. High Pull
2. Hang Snatch
3. Squat and Press
4. Bent-Over Alternating Row
5. Pushup
6. Core Row
ADVANCED BARBELL COMPLEX
1. Hang Muscle Snatch
2. Overhead Squat
3. Snatch Drop Balance
4. Overhead Lunge
5. Squat Hang Clean
6. Bent-Over Row and Good Morning

COMPLEX PAIRED EXERCISES (ADVANCED)

Plyometric Pushup (horiz push)	Squat Jump (knee bi)
Medicine Ball Drop (horiz push)	Split Box or Bench Jump (knee uni)
Medicine Ball Chest Pass	Ice Skater Jump (knee uni)
Medicine Ball Throw-Down (vert-horiz pull)	Medicine Ball Scoop
Box or Bench Jump (knee bi)	Romanian Deadlift Jump Shrug (hip bi)

2-DAY-PER-WEEK TRAINING SCHEDULE

If you choose the 2-day-per-week option, you will be using the full-body program shown on page 33, so try to space apart your workouts by at least 48 to 72 hours. This will ensure that all of our selected movements are trained twice each week. While it is possible to use the push-pull program as a 2-day-per-week workout, I would not recommend it, as there will be too much time (often a week or more) between the training of selected movements.

SAMPLE 2-DAY FULL-BODY WORKOUTS

DAY 1	DAY 2
Workout A	Workout B

3-DAY-PER-WEEK TRAINING SCHEDULE

Depending on your available time, a 3-day-per-week schedule can utilize either the full-body (page 33) or the push-pull (page 34) programs.

SAMPLE 3-DAY FULL-BODY WORKOUTS

DAY 1	DAY 2	DAY 3
Workout A	Workout B	Workout A
↓	↓	↓
(Next week)		
DAY 1	**DAY 2**	**DAY 3**
Workout B	Workout A	Workout B

SAMPLE 3-DAY PUSH-PULL WORKOUTS

DAY 1	DAY 2	DAY 3
Workout A1	Workout B1	Workout A2
↓	↓	↓
(Next week)		
DAY 1	**DAY 2**	**DAY 3**
Workout B2	Workout A1	Workout B1

4-DAY-PER-WEEK TRAINING SCHEDULE

For those of you who choose to use the 4-day training schedule, I recommend only using the push-pull program (page 34), as the full-body program done four times each week could lead to overtraining issues. This sequence can be done 4 days straight through or with a day off after your second workout.

SAMPLE 4-DAY PUSH-PULL WORKOUTS

DAY 1	DAY 2	DAY 3	DAY 4
Workout A1	Workout B1	Workout A2	Workout B2

HOW LONG SHOULD MY WORKOUTS TAKE TO COMPLETE?

Rather than being concerned about how long it takes to complete your sets, the length of your workouts is usually determined by how long you take between sets, socializing, changing equipment, etc. It is important to try to adhere to the prescribed rest periods between sets as this time period plays an important role in your training goals. It is also important to remember that changing weights and adjusting equipment should be factored into your rest times and that rest times start once your set is completed. Following are sample time breakdowns for both the full-body and push-pull workouts. Keep in mind that prescribed rest periods are longer in strength phases compared to hypertrophy phases and that many unilateral exercises take longer to complete due to the fact that each limb is often trained exclusively, thus creating double duration sets. The durations listed below are estimations based on average sessions. Individual workouts may run longer or shorter depending on choice of exercises, goals, and training experience.

SAMPLE PUSH-PULL PROGRAM DURATIONS

	WEEKS 1–3	WEEKS 4–6	WEEKS 7–9	WEEKS 10–12
	Power: 4 × 5	Power: 5 × 3	Power: 4 × 5	Power: 5 × 3
	Others: 4 × 10	Others: 4 × 6	Others: 4 × 8	Others: 4 × 4
EXAMPLE PUSH A1	WEEKS 1–3	WEEKS 4–6	WEEKS 7–9	WEEKS 10–12
Barbell Complex Warmup	30 reps	30 reps	30 reps	30 reps
Clean Pull	3–4 × 5	4–5 × 3	3–4 × 5	3–4 × 4
Front Squat	3–4 × 10	3–4 × 6	3–4 × 8	3–4 × 4
Dumbbell Bench Press	3–4 × 10	3–4 × 6	3–4 × 8	3–4 × 4
Push Press	3–4 × 10	3–4 × 6	3–4 × 8	3–4 × 4
Rotational/Bridge Core	3 × 10 + 3 min	3 × 10 + 3 min	3 × 10 + 3 min	3 × 10 + 3 min
	15–19 sets	14–18 sets	15–19 sets	15–19 sets
Approximate time to complete	**30–40 min**	**35–45 min**	**30–40 min**	**35–45 min**

SAMPLE FULL-BODY PROGRAM DURATIONS

	WEEKS 1–3	WEEKS 4–6	WEEKS 7–9	WEEKS 10–12
	Power: 4 × 5	Power: 5 × 3	Power: 4 × 5	Power: 5 × 3
	Others: 4 × 10	Others: 4 × 6	Others: 4 × 8	Others: 4 × 4

EXAMPLE FULL BODY B	WEEKS 1–3	WEEKS 4–6	WEEKS 7–9	WEEKS 10–12
Barbell Complex Warmup	30 reps	30 reps	30 reps	30 reps
Hang Power Clean	3–4 × 5	4–5 × 3	3–4 × 5	3–4 × 4
Stepup	3–4 × 10	3–4 × 6	3–4 × 8	3–4 × 4
Romanian Deadlift	3–4 × 10	3–4 × 6	3–4 × 8	3–4 × 4
Dumbbell Incline Bench Press	3–4 × 10	3–4 × 6	3–4 × 8	3–4 × 4
Standing Cable Row to Neck	3–4 × 10	3–4 × 6	3–4 × 8	3–4 × 4
Dumbbell Alternating Press	3–4 × 10	3–4 × 6	3–4 × 8	3–4 × 4
Lat Pulldown	3–4 × 10	3–4 × 6	3–4 × 8	3–4 × 4
Rotational/Bridge Core	3 × 10 + 3 min	3 × 10 + 3 min	3 × 10 + 3 min	3 × 10 + 3 min
	24–31 sets	25–32 sets	24–31 sets	24–31 sets
Approximate time to complete	**45–50 min**	**50–60 min**	**45–50 min**	**50–60 min**

HOW OFTEN SHOULD I CHANGE EXERCISES?

It is up to you. Since the Power Training program addresses all essential movements from both unilateral and bilateral performance, there will always be a variety of exercises to address each movement pattern. Varying exercises every week or two will afford you the opportunity to adjust by allowing you to perform each exercise for two to four workouts, thus making this a good option.

UNLOADING

When you work at high levels of intensity, it is often necessary to *unload*, or back off for a training session or more. The Power Training program is designed for 12-week cycles with four 3-week training blocks within each cycle. There are natural breaks every 3 weeks enabling you to unload at this point. I recommend that you incorporate an optional unloading at 6 weeks and a mandatory unloading at 12 weeks. This unloading can be as simple as using lighter weights for a workout or two, performing combination-style lifts, or excluding a workout or two completely. This will help both your body and your mind relax and rejuvenate to prepare for another block of training.

PART 3

THE POWER TRAINING EXERCISE MENU

THE BASICS OF MOVEMENT

In the chapters that follow you will find the *Men's Health* Power Training menu described exercise by exercise. But before we get into the actual exercises It is important to understand the basics of human movement and the planes in which we move. At right is an illustration of the three planes of movement: the sagittal plane, the frontal plane, and the transverse plane.

The *sagittal plane* involves movements of the body forward and backward. These are exercises like close squats and chinups. The *frontal plane* involves movements that occur laterally and includes exercises such as wide-grip lat pulldowns and shoulder presses. The *transverse plane* involves movements that occur around your body in a rotational fashion and includes exercises such as Russian core twists and bench presses. While I will make reference to these planes as I describe the exercises, it is most important to understand the menu movement categories. These will include vertical push and pull, horizontal push and pull, rotational, explosive (which can include any of the aforementioned movements), knee-dominant, hip-dominant, and bridging or core stabilization movements. Also note that oftentimes exercises will

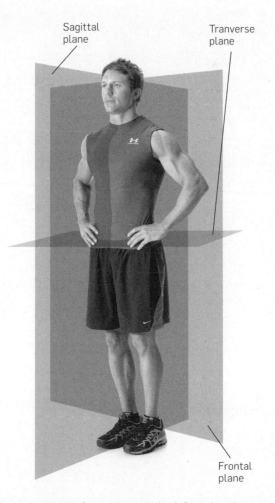

Sagittal plane

Tranverse plane

Frontal plane

The three planes of movement: sagittal, frontal, and transverse move in more than one plane. An example of this would be a drop lunge (page 71), which actually moves in all three of the planes.

When I refer to *horizontal,* I am talking about exercises that move horizontally when you are in a standing position. In other words, if you are lying down performing a bench press exercise, you are still working horizontally even though the bar is traveling vertically because if you stood up and performed this movement from the anatomical position, it would still be performing the same movement plane. When I refer to *vertical* movements, I am talking about exercises that move either up or down vertically when in a standing position. While the exercises on the lists address all possible movements on all planes, it is important to understand that both horizontal and vertical movements can and should involve exercises that move in all three planes when possible. In other words, you will want to make sure that you are not always performing chinups, which are a sagittal plane movement. Rather, from workout to workout, alternate to pullups, which are a frontal plane movement. The same will go for the horizontal movements. For instance, a close-grip bench press with elbows in is a horizontal push exercise that moves in your sagittal plane, while a traditional wider-grip bench press actually moves in your transverse plane. (It's critical to remember that if you understand movement planes, you will better understand how your muscles work during exercises. Muscles rarely work in just one plane. By choosing exercises that move on multiple planes, you will ensure that your muscles are working optimally.)

Since you are in control of selecting exercises from each category, it is my hope that your understanding of the planes and the movement categories will make this selection easier and more effective.

EXPLOSIVE EXERCISES

The *Men's Health* Power Training explosive exercise menu category is quite extensive. The reasoning here is that as you become more proficient with the basic exercises, you will be able to further challenge yourself by moving to more difficult variations. As you can see in the figure at right, it is difficult to pinpoint one specific muscle group that will be targeted during these exercises. As I mention in Chapter 2, it is the rapid quadruple extension of the ankles, knees, hips, and even lower back that enables us to generate a great deal of power during these exercises. If you recall the information in Chapter 1 regarding power versus strength, you will remember that it is the speed of these movements that is so important to the production and development of power. If I was to name the single important menu category that is generally sadly neglected, it would be this one. Most trainees don't see the importance of incorporating these types of exercises in their training programs.

While many people are somewhat intimidated by the technical aspects of the Olympic-style lifts, I will show you several variations that even beginners can successfully learn (and handle) in minutes. Every one of these explosive exercises meets every criterion in what qualifies as the perfect functional exercise (as described in Chapter 2):

• Performed unsupported—on your feet

• Uses free weights

• Explosive

• Multiple-joint—compound exercise

The exercises are listed from beginner to advanced. It is perfectly fine to stay in the basic category indefinitely. In fact, I would not recommend progressing to the more technical exercises without proper hands-on coaching.

Explosive exercises target the calves, hamstrings, quadriceps, glutes, lower back, upper back, and shoulders.

47

SQUAT JUMP

This is one of the simplest ways to teach the explosive training. While it doesn't involve very much upper-body movement, it is a great way to target powerful ankle, knee, and hip extension.

Set your feet in a squatting base, as if you are about to squat with a heavy load, with hands behind your head. Descend into a parallel position and then drive up as high as possible, making sure to consciously push as hard as you can through your ankles, knees, and hips. Upon landing, attempt to absorb the load of the jump by landing on the front half of your feet and then sinking back onto your heels as the hips descend into the next squat.

Tip: Using dumbbells will allow you to add the shrug component and often forces your body to extend more at the lower back to move the load, thus making this movement very similar to the Olympic-style lifts.

You can perform these by setting your feet and taking a breath between jumps or do them continuously, sort of like a spring. Start off by performing these with no weights, using only your body weight, and then progress to the bar (placed behind your neck) or light dumbbells held at arm's length. When the load gets too heavy to perform a decent jump, you'll need to lessen the weight.

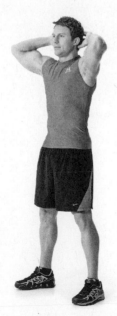
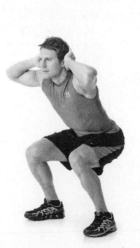
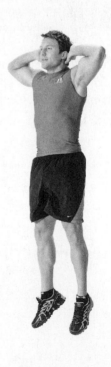

HANG JUMP SHRUG

This exercise is basically the beginning of all the Olympic-style lifts from the hang, or power, position. This, along with all the exercises preceded by "hang," will begin from the power position described on page 51. These exercises are all great total body exercises that will help you generate and develop a lot of power.

Start by holding the bar with a pronated grip and your hands approximately shoulder-width apart. From a standing position, lower the bar to the top of your kneecaps by *slightly* bending your knees and pushing your hips back. You need to keep your lower back flat, your eyes up, and you should look like you are leaning forward "looking out a window" rather than "sitting in a chair."

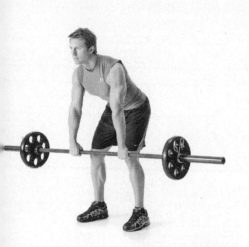

From this position, push into the ground as hard as possible to extend your torso and jump off the ground. Make sure to forcefully shrug your shoulders to aid in the movement of the load. Your arms should be kept almost completely straight during the entire movement. As you land, try to land with your feet *flat*. I know this sounds funny, but by landing flat-footed with your knees bent and hips back, you place the heavy load onto your hips rather than your knees (which would occur if we landed on the front half of your feet). After landing, reset yourself into the lowered power position before starting the next repetition.

This exercise can be done using dumbbells as well.

CLEAN AND SNATCH PULLS

This is a very basic, yet effective power exercise and one that can be learned rather quickly. The bar starts on the floor with these exercises. Using a larger plate like a 45-pound Olympic plate (on both ends of the bar), you should have no problem getting into the starting position. However, if you are using a smaller plate, like a 25- or a 10-pound plate, the bar will most likely be a bit too low if it is sitting on the ground. If this is the case, prior to the start of the exercise, lift the weights off the floor, to about mid-shin height.

CLEAN PULL

Hold the bar using a pronated grip approximately shoulder-width apart. The bar is on the floor (bar approximately mid-shin height), and close to touching your shin, your hips are down, feet flat and shoulders tall. Your back should not be rounded at all. Forcefully drive into the ground to pull the bar off the floor. You are not pulling with your arms, but rather with your hips on this exercise, so make sure your arms stay extended throughout the movement. As the bar comes off the ground, try to keep the angle of your back constant. Your legs basically start to straighten to bring your body up. As the bar begins to cross the knees, you should be in the perfect power position just like the jump shrug. Pull and shrug as hard as you can in an attempt to make the bar move as fast as possible.

Tip: *The key to a successful pull from the floor is to not let your hips rise faster than your shoulders as this will cause your lower back to round and increase your risk of injury.*

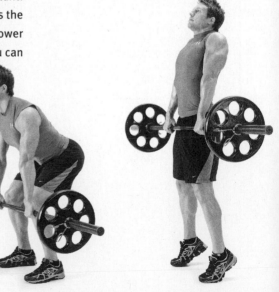

THE POWER POSITION

This is a very important position to become familiar with when performing the power exercises. It is in this position (often referred to as the second-pull position or the hang position with the Olympic lifts) that we will generate the most power. Setting yourself in a solid position will assure stability, decrease your chance of injury, and increase your ability to generate valuable power.

✓ Set your feet in what I call a *jumping base*; this is the base you would use if you were to try to jump as high as possible.

✓ Slightly bend your knees.

✓ Keeping your back arched and shoulders back, slide your hands down your thighs until they are even with your knees. This movement should be initiated by pushing your hips back and bending at the hips rather than at the knees.

✓ At this point you should look like you are leaning way forward, almost as if you are looking out of a window and trying to counterbalance with your hips so that you don't fall out.

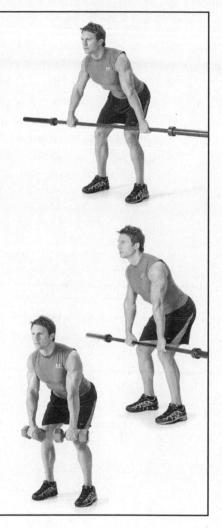

SNATCH PULL

This exercise is identical to the clean pull with the exception of the grip width. You will be using a snatch grip, which is quite a bit wider than shoulder width. A quick way to determine the width of your individual snatch grip is to pick up an empty bar and pull it up until your upper arms are parallel with the floor. Looking in a mirror, place your grip where your elbows make a right angle in this position. Due to this wider grip, you will have to bend down farther to get into the starting position when doing snatch pulls.

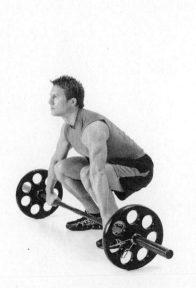

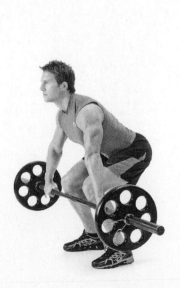

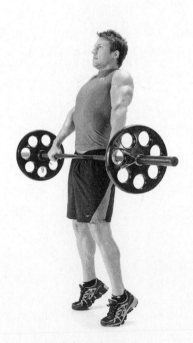

CLEAN AND SNATCH HIGH PULLS

Tip: *Your arms should stay extended as long as possible; the bar will be traveling past your thighs and the shrug movement should precede the arm pulling.*

This is a continuation of the pulls described earlier. Unlike the clean and snatch pulls, this exercise includes pulling with your arms to finish the movement.

CLEAN HIGH PULL

Perform a standard pull. As the bar reaches your thighs, continue by pulling your elbows up toward the ceiling. The end of the pull should have you in a position with your elbows high, hips extended, up on your toes. This is a great preliminary exercise to the power clean or hang power clean.

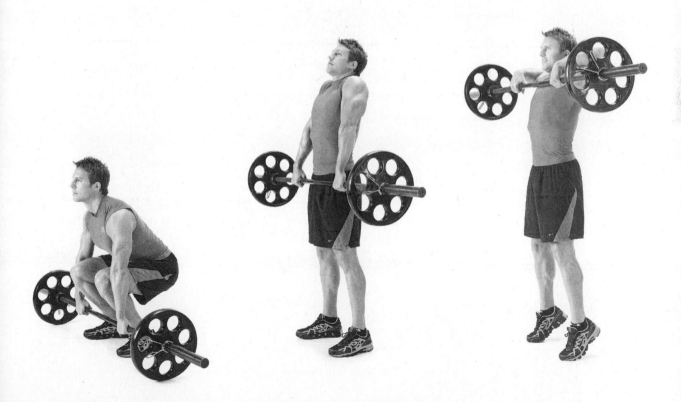

SNATCH HIGH PULL

Just like the clean high pull, perform a snatch pull and keep pulling vertically with your arms. You will not be able to pull the bar as high due to the wider grip. This is a great preliminary exercise to the power snatch or hang power snatch.

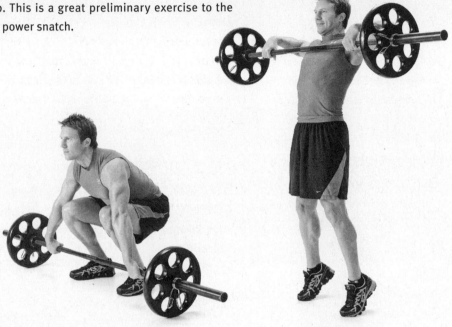

"WHEN THE ELBOWS BEND, THE POWER ENDS!"

This is a phrase I use to emphasize the fact that you really need to exaggerate the movement of your hips and the shrugging of your shoulders when doing these pull exercises. Once you start pulling with your arms, you will essentially "turn off" the power switch in your hips and legs. Therefore, the arm pull needs to come at the very last moment of these high pulls or even later when you attempt to do the actual power cleans or snatches.

Remember, successfully completing these lifts depends on the rapid and powerful quadruple extension that I described earlier. You don't want to compromise the effectiveness of this movement by pulling with your arms too soon.

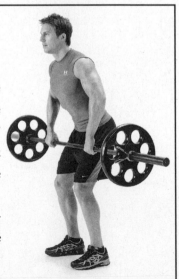

Tip: *There is an audible cue that you should hear when doing this exercise. The bar should be caught at your shoulders at the same time you hear your feet hit the ground (from the sliding out). You can also perform this exercise with dumbbells. I suggest catching the dumbbells so that the flat side of the dumbbell is resting squarely on your shoulders.*

POWER CLEANS AND POWER SNATCHES

Once you become comfortable with the pulls, you can begin to play with the actual power-clean and power-snatch exercises. The term power *is used in these exercises to describe the position of your body when you "catch" the weights either at your shoulders (clean) or overhead (snatch). Your knees will be bent and your body will be in about a quarter-squat position with your feet flat and hips back.*

Keep in mind that the fundamentals used in the pulls will still apply. All we are doing is adding to the equation; we are not changing anything. The tendency is to use your arms more on these exercises, but this will result In poor form. There is a point in a high pull when the bar will reach its highest point. At this time, the load will encounter zero gravity. This is the fraction of a second when the bar is neither rising nor falling—it is basically weightless. It is at this point that we attempt to catch the bar.

HANG POWER CLEAN

Start with the bar in the hang, or power, position resting in front of your quads. From here perform a high pull. When the bar is at its highest point, your body should be in a fully extended position (up on your toes). To catch the bar at your shoulders, slide your feet out laterally to a catching base, which is a few inches wider than your pulling or jumping base. Simultaneously slide your feet out, drop your hips, and rotate your elbows down and around the bar. Make sure to rotate your elbows *around the bar* rather than moving the bar around your arms.

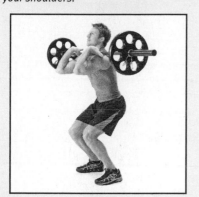

The bar will land on your shoulders. Open your hands slightly so the load of the bar rests on the front of your shoulders. Regrip the bar and lower back to the hang position for the next rep.

POWER CLEAN

The power clean is simply the aforementioned exercise with the addition of the first pull. Start with the bar on the ground (or at mid shin if using smaller plates than 45s). Just as with the clean or high pulls, attempt to maintain the starting back angle as your knees unbend to raise the bar to your knees. From here, continue with a hang clean.

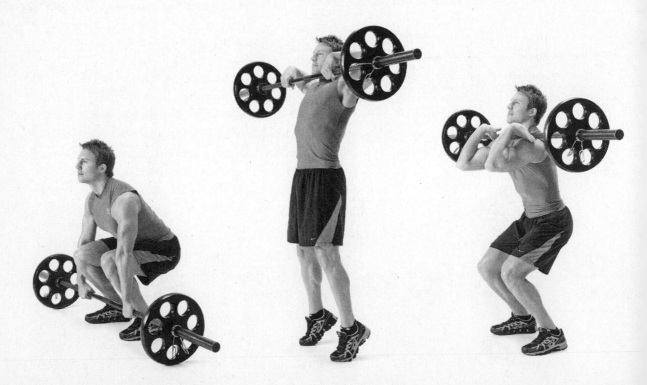

HANG POWER SNATCH

The snatch is more difficult because you need quite a bit of balance and flexibility to properly execute this exercise. Remember that with the exception of your grip and where the bar is caught (overhead versus at the shoulders), the fundamentals are the same as with the hang power clean. Start with the bar in the hang, or power, position, hands out to your snatch grip. Follow the same sequence of the snatch high pull. At the bar's highest point, "pull yourself under the bar" by dropping your hips, sliding your feet out to the catching base, and rotating your elbows under the bar.

You need to forcefully drive your arms into an extended position so that the bar is stable overhead. Timing is crucial because you need to lock out your elbows as your feet hit the ground in the catching base. The bar will finish overhead, slightly behind your ears.

Tip: *Be careful when lowering the bar to your shoulders as the wide grip puts your shoulders in a more vulnerable position. You can also perform this exercise with dumbbells. When catching the weight overhead, make sure the dumbbells are directly above your shoulders so you do not lose control of the load.*

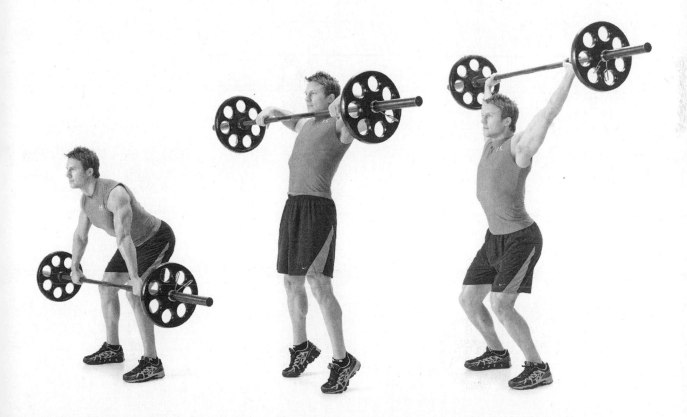

THE MUSCLE SNATCH

This is a great preparatory exercise for the snatch exercise. Using a light load, start with the bar in the hang position and hands in a snatch grip. Use your hips to perform a snatch high pull. At the top of the pull, continue by rotating your hands under the bar and pressing the weight out overhead. You will not shift your feet or drop your hips to catch in a power position.

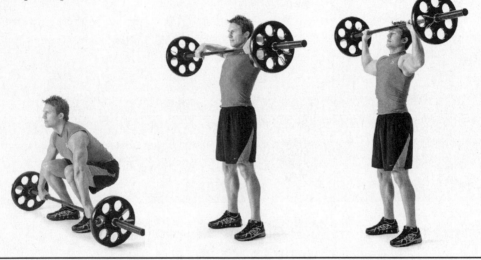

POWER SNATCH

Like the power clean, the power snatch is simply the hang snatch done with the addition of the first pull. Start with the bar on the ground (or at mid shin if using smaller plates than 45s). Just as with the clean or high pulls, attempt to maintain the starting back angle as your knees bend to raise the bar to the knees. From here you are simply performing a hang snatch.

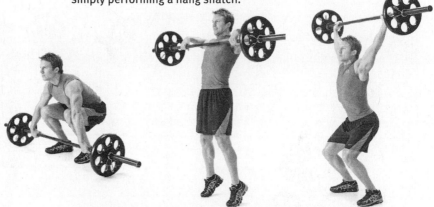

NARROW-GRIP POWER SNATCH

This exercise is identical to the power snatch but uses a grip similar to the power cleans. This grip makes the exercise a bit more difficult due to the longer pull, but is easier on the shoulders, especially when lowering the weight after completing each rep.

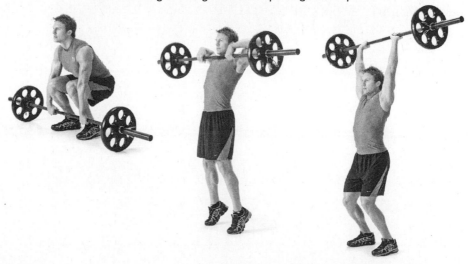

ONE-ARM DUMBBELL SNATCH

This is one of my favorite exercises and it is also easier to master than the traditional snatch. You can perform these from a hang position or from the floor. Holding a dumbbell either at your knees or on the floor, perform a high pull, making sure to follow all the fundamentals mentioned earlier. At the dumbbell's highest point, slide into the catching base, drop your hips, and drive under the weight by rotating under the dumbbell, and quickly extend your elbow. The weight should be over the top of your shoulder and your torso should be erect rather than tilted.

Tip: If using heavier loads, bring the dumbbell back down to your shoulders with both hands before lowering it back down to the starting position.

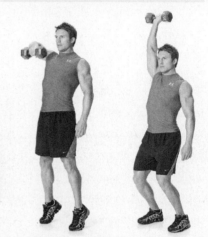
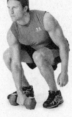

CATCHING THE WEIGHTS

I have already talked about the power position with your feet in a jumping base. I want to now address the "catch" during the power cleans and power snatches.

During the course of the quadruple extension, your feet will physically leave the ground prior to catching the weight either at the shoulders or overhead. It is important to make sure you have a stable base of support for catching the weight. This is where you will have to shift your feet out slightly into what I call your *catching base* with knees bent and hips back.

The other alternative catching base is called a *split catch*, as shown in the photos at right, where you will split one leg out in front of the other to create a stable base, with your front leg bent and your back leg slightly bent and feet about hip-width apart.

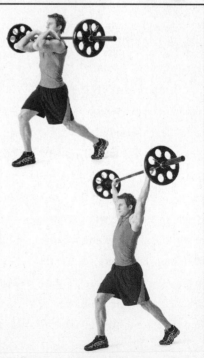

KNEE-DOMINANT EXERCISES

This group of exercises is categorized based on similarity of movement and targeted muscle groups. These knee-dominant exercises are all initiated by an extension of the knee joint, which in turn leads to additional extension at the hip joint. The simple concept that I use to help remember these exercises is that all of these movements begin by using a "pushing" force into the ground to extend your knee and hip joints. Because of this, these exercises are also grouped into the "push" exercises when using a "push-pull" split routine.

Remember that it's important to train these knee-dominant exercises both bilaterally and unilaterally to assure muscle balance and improve stability. So you will use a bilateral exercise one workout and a unilateral exercise the next. In addition, you should try to use as many of the exercises in the menu as possible as some will primarily train in a straight-ahead or sagittal-plane movement while others will elicit more of a lateral- or frontal-plane muscle movement. All of the exercises in the knee-dominant menu are closed kinetic chain movements, which means that the force is applied into the ground, rather than into the weight. This makes them extremely functional exercises.

SET YOUR CORE!

"Set your core" is a phrase I borrowed from Chris Doyle, strength and conditioning coach at the University of Iowa. I use it when telling people to ready their bodies for any heavy lifts performed while standing (i.e., power cleans, push presses, front squats, and so forth). All this means is to take in a chest full of air and squeeze down prior to performing a repetition. This will activate your core muscles and ensure that your spine is being supported throughout the exercise.

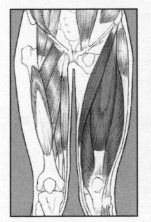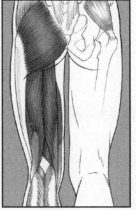

Knee-dominant exercises target the quadriceps, hamstrings, and gluteals.

61

FRONT SQUAT

Remember that I have already labeled these as the "king of all lower-body exercises" (see Chapter 3) so I definitely recommend becoming proficient at them. In addition, if you intend to become proficient at the Olympic-style lifts like the power clean or hang clean, I would suggest that you use the "catch" grip when performing these.

Using one of the grips pictured at right, rest the bar on the front of your shoulders. The bar should be in contact with your neck, with your elbows held high in front to keep the bar in place. Set your core by filling your chest with air and maintaining a tight, vertical torso. Descend as deep as possible by pushing your hips back, keeping your shin angle the same as your back angle to keep your heels flat. Drive upward and exhale as you pass the halfway point during the ascent.

Tip: *Try using a hands-free position with light weight, with your arms held out front and the bar resting on your shoulders with no grip support. This will help you get used to resting the weight on your shoulders and keeping your torso erect.*

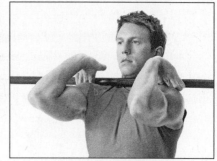

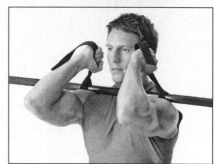

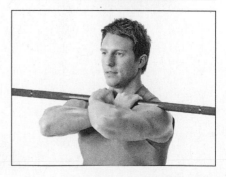

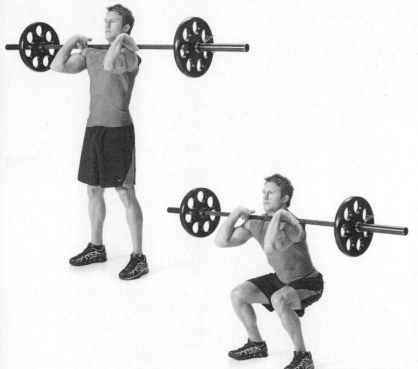

BACK SQUAT

While I believe that back squats can be a key component to your program, I often see drastic changes in form, loads, and technique during their performance that make me an even bigger believer. The general changes that I see are too much torso forward lean and increases in load, which often compromise the depth of the squat. However, if you are able to keep your torso erect and maintain the same depth as your front squats, more power to you!

Place the bar behind your neck and rest it on your trapezius to avoid direct contact with your cervical vertebrae. As with the front squats, set your core and maintain an erect torso as you descend as deep as possible, making sure to keep your heels flat, hips slightly back, and your knees behind your toes. Drive upward and exhale as you pass the halfway point during the ascent.

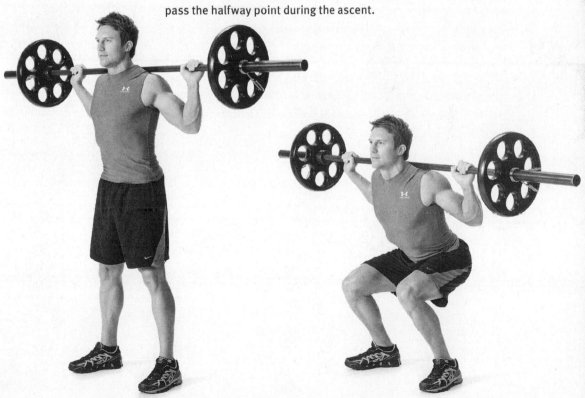

OVERHEAD SQUAT

I'm not going to kid you. Overhead squats are a very tough exercise, but their benefits are tremendous. Not only do they target all the same muscle groups as the other squats, but they also tax the core and help develop tremendous balance. The loads do not have to be very high with this exercise, as the position of the bar will make just about any load seem difficult.

Using a wide (snatch) grip, start with the bar resting behind your neck. Set your feet into a good squatting base and extend the bar overhead. You will need to place the bar slightly behind your ears and retracting your scapula (shoulder blades) to maintain solid stability in this position. Focus your eyes outward (not down) while keeping your chest high and shoulders back. Maintaining a solid arch in your lower back, try to keep your torso as vertical as possible (you won't be able to maintain as erect a torso as with your front or back squats, and this is okay).

Descend as deep as possible, making sure to keep your heels flat and hips pushed back for balance. Keep your core set, drive upward, and exhale as you pass the halfway point during the ascent.

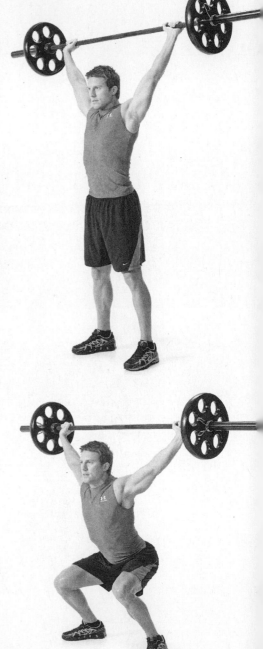

SPLIT SQUAT

A great change-up to your traditional squat base setting where your feet are even, split squats enable you to train bilaterally with a very unfamiliar base of support. Note that you will have to perform all of the reps with each leg in the forward position. In other words, a set of 10 would be 10 with your right foot forward, then 10 with your left.

Place the bar on either the front of the shoulders like a front squat or behind your neck. Place one foot well out in front of the other in a staggered position. Set your core and maintain an erect torso as you descend as deep as possible with the front heel firmly on the floor and the rear heel slightly raised. Attempt to push with the back leg as much as possible. Drive upward and exhale as you pass the half-way point during the ascent.

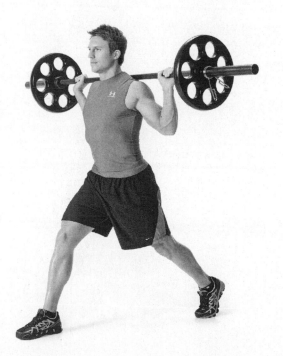
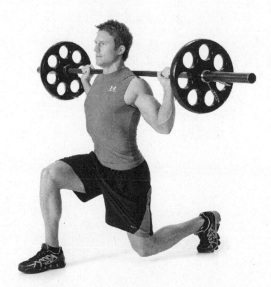

SIDE SQUAT

This lateral movement squat looks similar to a lunge. The big difference is that your feet stay firmly in place during the entire exercise. This is a great movement to develop strength in all three planes of movement!

Place the bar behind your neck. Set your feet wider than you would for your front or back squats and point your toes out slightly. Set your core, and keeping your chest up and shoulders back, move to the right and down, pushing your hips back to keep your heels flat. It is normal to lean slightly forward as you descend in this exercise. Drive upward and exhale as you approach the upright position. Immediately repeat this movement to the left. This is 1 repetition.

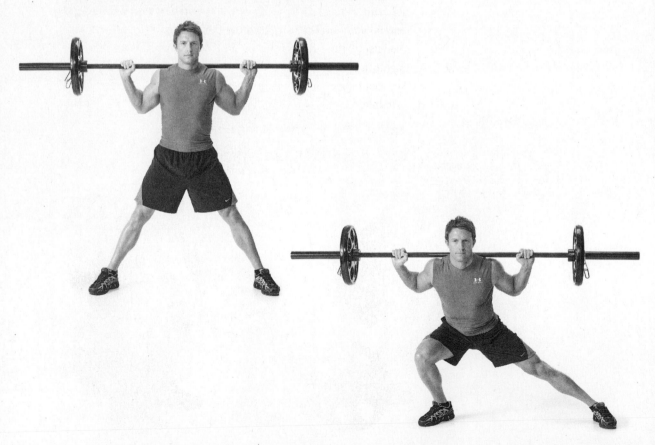

CLEAN-GRIP DEADLIFT

Yes indeed, I have included deadlifts in the knee-dominant category. Why, you may ask? Well, because I can't see a whole lot of difference between a traditional deadlift and a squat. With the exception of where the bar is in relation to your body, everything else should look almost identical if this exercise is done correctly. I still consider this a pushing exercise since the force is applied into the ground to initiate knee and hip extension.

With the bar on the ground, grip it using a pronated shoulder-width grip (similar to what you would use to perform a power clean). Set your torso tall and raise your shoulders up as you extend your arms and drive your hips down. Set your core in this position and forcefully drive your feet into the ground as you raise your shoulders and extend your knees. Exhale as you pass the halfway point of this exercise. Return the bar to the ground by reversing these movements in a controlled manner, making sure to bend your knees and set your hips back on the descent, keeping your torso as vertical as possible.

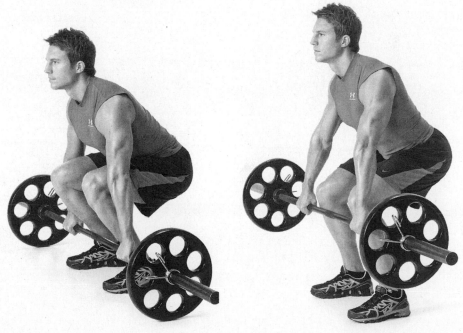

FORWARD LUNGE

These are traditionally some of the toughest lunges around. Not only do you have to decelerate a weight that is moving forward, but you also need to generate enough force to return the load back to the starting position.

Place the bar either on the front of your shoulders like a front squat (bar position shown at right) or behind your neck. Stand with your feet even and at about hip width. Step one foot forward as far as possible, landing heel first. Descend until the back knee almost touches the ground and immediately drive upward and back to the starting position. Set your core at the starting position and exhale as you pass the halfway point during the ascent.

Tip: Many of the knee-dominant exercises can be performed with the bar placed in a front squat position, making the exercise more difficult.

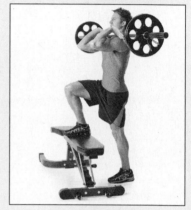

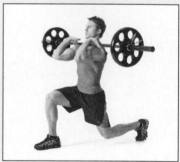

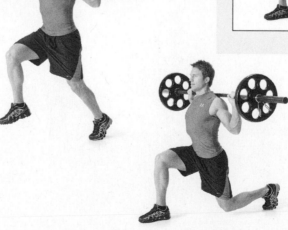

REVERSE LUNGE

Reverse lunges are not as difficult as the forward lunge so you can usually use slightly heavier loads. The biggest difference between this movement and the forward lunge is the work distance traveled and the manner in which force is applied (backward in a forward lunge and vertical in a reverse lunge).

Place the bar either on the front of your shoulders like a front squat or behind your neck. Stand with your feet even and at about hip width. Set your core and step one foot backward as far as possible, placing the ball of your foot on the ground. Descend until your back knee nearly touches the ground and immediately drive upward and back to the starting position. Exhale as you pass the halfway point during the ascent.

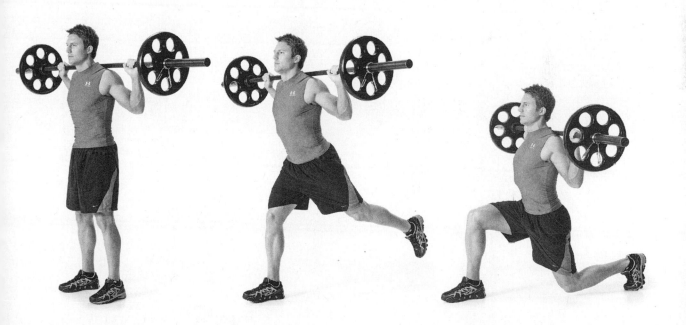

SIDE LUNGE

This is a great lunge variation that enables you to train in a lateral fashion. Unlike a side squat, the side lunge requires you to travel out and back to the original starting position, thus keeping the lunging movement pattern.

Place the bar either on the front of your shoulders like a front squat or behind your neck. Set your core and stand with your feet close together. Step sideways with your right foot out as far as possible, landing flat-footed, and sink into a deep side lunge position. Forcefully push back up to the starting position. Repeat on the left side. This is 1 repetition. Exhale as you approach the initial starting position.

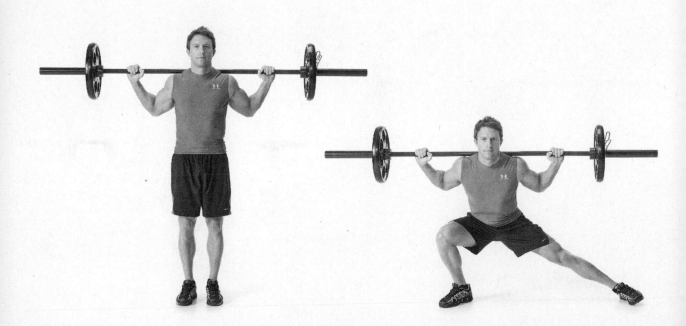

DROP LUNGE

This is one of my all-time favorite lunge variations because it allows action on all three planes of movement. I especially like the rotational movement at the hip. This exercise is sometimes called a curtsy lunge, but I don't think most guys feel comfortable "curtsying."

Place the bar either on the front of your shoulders like a front squat or behind your neck. Set your core and stand with your feet even and at about hip width. Step your left foot back and across the opposite leg. Try to reach as far back and as wide as possible as you sink into a deep lunge. Place the ball of your foot on the ground. Descend down until your back knee nearly touches the ground and immediately drive upward to return to the starting position. Exhale as you approach the starting position. Your front foot should stay pointed straight ahead and the bar should move side to side with little to no rotation.

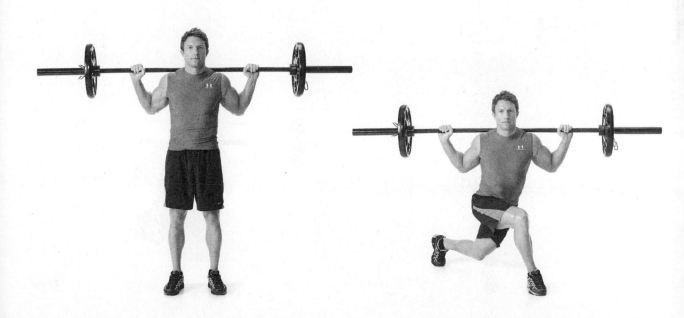

STEPUP

This is a tremendous unilateral knee-dominant exercise that allows you to see strength imbalances almost immediately. I would suggest a bench or box no higher than 18 inches or a height that allows your hip angle to exceed no more than 90 degrees when one foot is on top of the bench.

Place the bar either on the front of the shoulders like a front squat or behind your neck. Stand with your feet even and at about hip width facing the bench. Step your right foot on top of the bench and drive upward until your other foot is able to step up on top of the bench. Make sure to extend all the way up using only the working leg. Do not place your other foot on the bench until you reach this point. Pause at the top and lower your left foot back down to the ground, maintaining control so that it lands softly on the ground. Do all the repetitions while keeping your right foot on top of the bench. Do not take it off the bench until you complete your reps. Now repeat with your other leg. This will complete 1 set. I use this technique because it isolates one limb very well and makes the same leg work concentrically and eccentrically in a back-to-back fashion. Set your core at the starting position and exhale as you approach the top of the bench.

Tip: To increase the intensity of your stepups, try holding the bar in the front position.

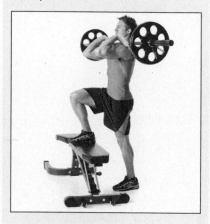

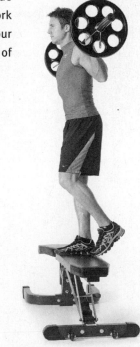

LATERAL STEPUP

Like the traditional stepup, the lateral stepup will expose weaknesses right away. Similar to the drop lunge, this exercise has a tremendous rotational component to its movement because you will be addressing all three planes once again.

Place the bar either on the front of your shoulders like a front squat or behind your neck. Stand with your feet even and at about hip width on the left side of a bench or box. Step your outside (left) foot across your body and on top of the bench while attempting to keep your toe pointed straight ahead. Step all the way up to the top of the bench and place both feet down. Pause and step off the other side with your near foot (right). Do not crossover step on the way down. Repeat on the other side. This is 1 repetition. As with the drop lunge, the bar should move side to side with little to no rotation. Set your core at the starting position and exhale as you approach the top of the bench.

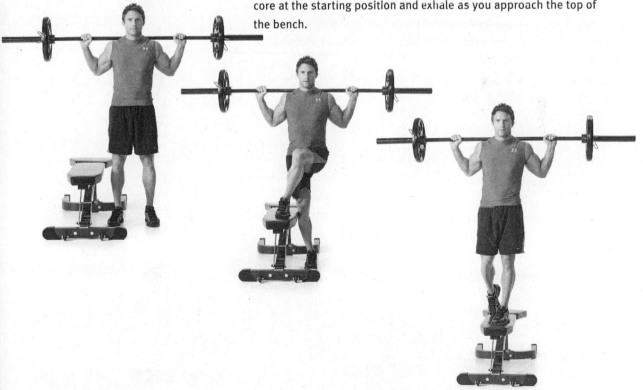

BULGARIAN SPLIT SQUAT

This is another great unilateral exercise that allows you to use a good amount of load once you become proficient at it. Unlike the regular split squat where you attempt to push close to 50 percent of the load with the rear leg, the Bulgarian split squat uses the rear leg only for balance as the forward leg does the bulk of the work. This is a great balance developer as your rear foot will be placed on top of a box or bench as your legs are positioned in a wide split.

Place the bar either on the front of your shoulders like a front squat or behind your neck. Place one foot well out in front of the other in a staggered position with your rear foot placed firmly on top of a bench or box no higher than 18 inches. Set your core and maintain an erect torso as you descend as deep as possible with your front heel firmly on the floor. You should feel a stretch in your rear leg's hip flexor region as you descend. Drive upward and exhale as you pass the halfway point during the ascent. Complete all the repetitions with one leg, then switch to the other to complete the same number of reps. This is 1 set.

Tip: As with lunges and stepups, try holding the bar in the front position to increase intensity.

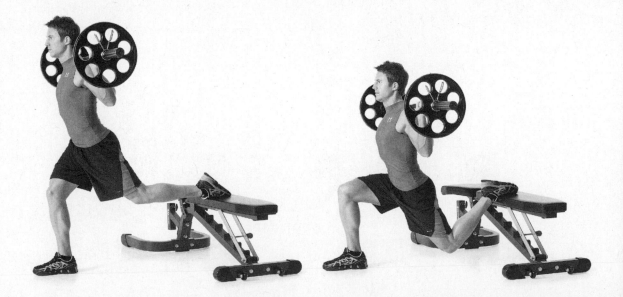

BULGARIAN SPLIT DEADLIFT

It's actually quite amazing how an exercise that looks almost identical to the Bulgarian split squat can feel so incredibly different. You will find that the same load used in this deadlift variation will seem much heavier. As with the Bulgarian split squat, you will use your rear leg only for balance as your forward leg does the bulk of the work.

Place the bar on the ground in front of you as you position yourself in a wide split with your rear foot on top of a bench or box. Move the bar close enough to your body so that it almost makes contact with the front of your shin. As with a traditional deadlift, keep your hips down, your chest up and shoulders back. Drive into the ground while keeping your arms locked to pull the bar off the floor. Think about simultaneously extending your knee as your shoulders rise rather than extending your knee first and then raising your shoulders. Emphasize lowering the weight back to the floor by bending your knee, dropping your hips and controlling the weight during the descent with your front leg and *not* your lower back. Set your core and maintain an erect torso as you ascend, exhaling as you approach the top of the movement. Complete all the repetitions with one leg, then switch to the other to complete the same number of reps. This is 1 set.

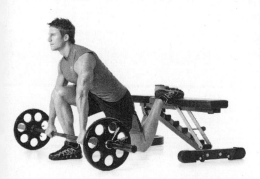

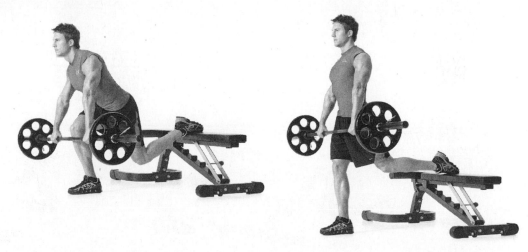

SINGLE-LEG SQUATS

If the front squat is the king of all lower-body exercises, the single-leg squat is a very close second. These tend to be one of the "not likely to be seen performed in your gym" exercises. That's not because they aren't extremely effective, mind you. It's really because they are one of the most difficult exercises known to man! Don't shy away from these if you are unable to complete a full single-leg or "pistol" squat, though I will show you several "build-up" options. As my friend and fellow strength coach Mike Boyle says, "I describe this as <u>real</u> lower-body strength: the ability to move your own body weight while stabilizing in two planes (frontal/transverse) and moving in one (sagittal)." I say show me a guy in the gym doing sets of full one-legged body-weight squats and I'll show you a strong individual. I will describe the different levels of these single-leg squats below.

LEVEL 1: SINGLE-LEG BENCH GETUP

Sitting on a bench with one foot on the ground and the other in the air, reach your arms forward and rock forward as you move to a standing position from one foot. As you get stronger, use less arm and torso movement. Repeat with your other leg.

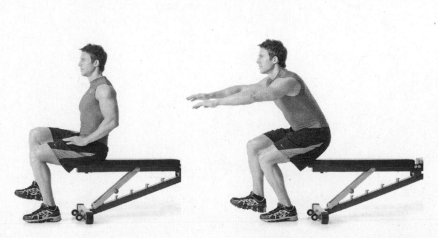
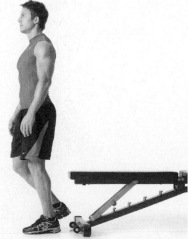

LEVEL 2: CROUCHING SINGLE-LEG SQUAT

Standing on one leg and bending the opposite, push your hips back as you attempt to lower your knee to the ground. Counterbalance by reaching your arms forward.

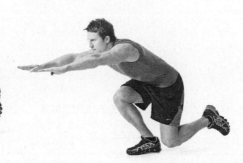

LEVEL 3: PARTIAL SINGLE-LEG SQUAT USING A BENCH OR BOX FOR DEPTH

Stand with a standard bench placed approximately one foot behind you. Extend one leg out in front of your body at about a 45-degree angle. Push your hips back and keep your heel flat on the floor as you descend until you feel your upper hamstring touch the bench and drive upward to the starting position. Reach your arms forward to aid with your balance.

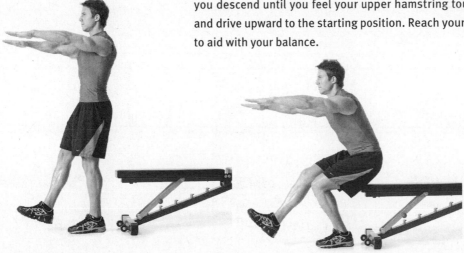

LEVEL 4: PARTIAL SINGLE-LEG SQUAT STANDING ON A BENCH

Stand on top of a bench with your inside foot close to the outer edge and let your outside leg hang down. Pushing your hips back and reaching your arms forward, try to lower your outside leg until it touches the floor. Rise back to the starting position. Try holding a 5- or 10-pound weight in your hands (in a reached-out forward position) as you descend, as this will help to counterbalance the load of your body.

LEVEL 5: SINGLE-LEG SQUAT STANDING ON A BENCH

Same as level 4 above, but with a greater range of motion.

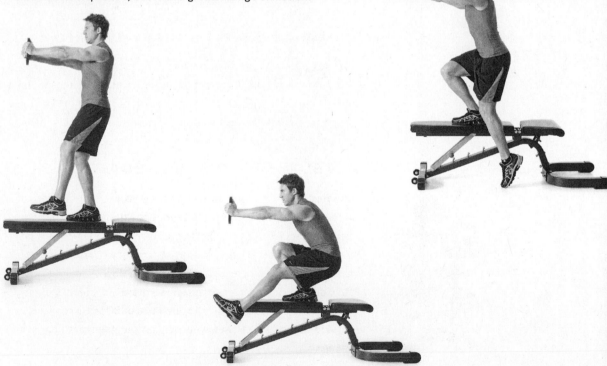

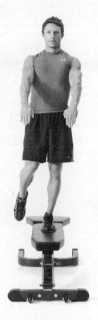

LEVEL 6: SINGLE-LEG SQUAT (LATERAL)

Same as the one-leg squat while standing on a bench except you will add some lateral movement to this already difficult exercise. Stand with your left foot on the bench and closest to the left side of the bench. Lower yourself and attempt to touch your right toe on the ground behind you. Repeat the set on the other leg.

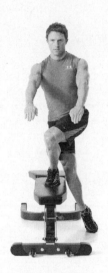

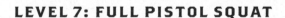

LEVEL 7: FULL PISTOL SQUAT

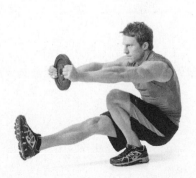

Standing on the ground, extend one leg up to approximately 45 degrees. Lower yourself into a full squat position keeping the lifted leg off the floor, ending parallel to the floor (should resemble a pistol gun) with your arms extended out in front of you. Make sure your heel stays flat on the ground the entire time. Rise back to the starting position. You can make this exercise more difficult by standing on an unstable surface such as an Airex pad or BOSU Ball or even by crossing your arms in front of your torso rather than reaching them forward.

HIP-DOMINANT EXERCISES

This category of exercises involves the extension of the hip with little to no knee extension. These hip-dominant exercises are initiated by a contraction of the hamstrings, glutes, and lower back to extend the hip. Since this movement is more of a pull than a push, it is placed with the "pulling" exercises if you are using a push-pull split routine. Like the knee-dominant exercises, it is important to train these hip-dominant exercises both bilaterally and unilaterally to assure muscle balance and improve stability. Training these exercises unilaterally can often be quite difficult and will take some getting used to, but the benefits will be well worth the work.

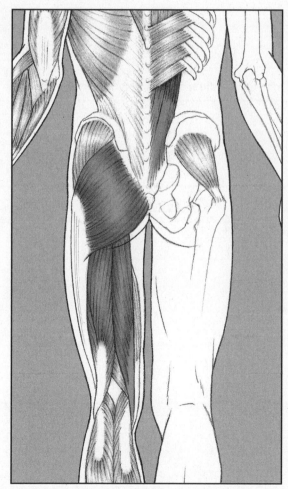

Hip-dominant exercises target the hamstrings, gluteals, and spinal erectors.

81

GOOD MORNING

A tremendous hip-dominant exercise, good mornings require much less load than many of the other listed exercises simply due to the location of the load during the exercise.

Rest the bar behind the neck, on the trapezius area of the shoulders. Keep your head up, shoulders back, and lower back *arched* during the entire exercise movement. Inhale prior to the start. Begin the movement by pushing your hips back as your chest lowers toward the ground. The range of motion in this exercise is dictated by your hamstring flexibility. Basically, you will move down as far as possible, attempting to get as close to parallel as possible while keeping your back arched. Once this arch begins to disappear, immediately start the upward phase of the exercise. Remember to keep your knees slightly bent during the entire exercise; this helps avoid hyperextending the knee.

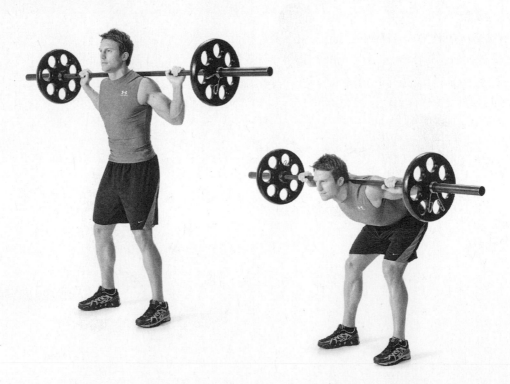

SEATED GOOD MORNING

This is a great exercise and one that allows someone with good flexibility to make a good morning a bit tougher.

As with the standard good morning, rest the bar behind your neck, on the trapezius. Keep your head up, shoulders back, and lower back *arched* during the entire exercise movement. While sitting on a bench, extend your legs in front of your body with knees slightly bent and heels on the floor. Lower your chest toward the bench while looking up to prevent the lower back from losing its arch. At your full range of motion, contract the posterior chain muscles to drive the weight back up to the starting position. This exercise tends to target the lower back more than the standard good morning.

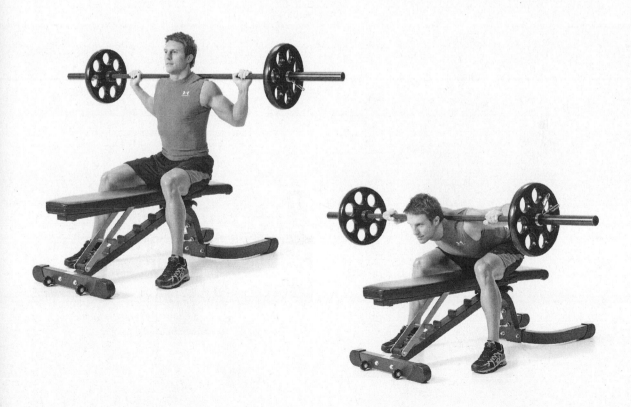

ZERCHER GOOD MORNING

One of my personal favorite exercises, this is a simple variation of the good morning movement with the difference being the location of the bar load.

Wrap a bar with a towel or pad to protect your arms. Pick up the bar by placing it in the crease of your elbow, just below the biceps. Maintain the same posture as the standard good morning and keep your hands in contact with your chin as you move downward.

Tip: *Don't place the bar directly in the elbow crease; rather, squeeze it between your forearm and biceps muscles as this will cause less discomfort. Maintain the same breathing pattern as the standard good morning.*

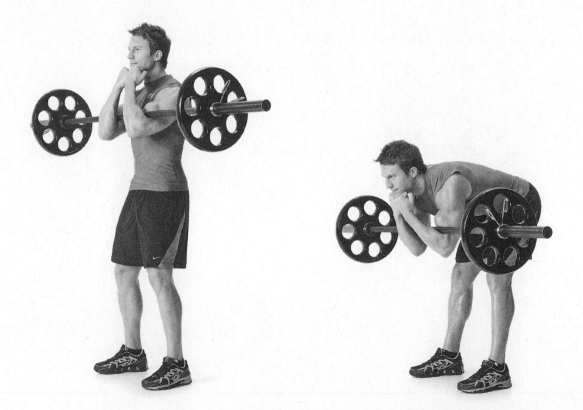

ROMANIAN DEADLIFT

Tip: *Push your hips backward to start the movement, so much, in fact, that your toes may start to rise as the weight is lowered.*

Probably our number-one hip-dominant exercise simply due to its similarity in movement patterns to many of the Olympic-style lifts. Unlike a traditional clean-grip deadlift, this Romanian deadlift (or stiff-leg dead, as some call it) is initiated by the hips rather than the knees. I teach these with the same posture as a good morning. We can also add quite a bit more load when executing this exercise compared to the good mornings.

Stand and hold the bar with a pronated grip, at arm's length. Feet are shoulder-width apart and knees slightly bent. Keep your head up, shoulders back, and lower back arched as you lower the bar toward the floor while keeping your knees slightly bent. As with the good mornings, your range of motion is dictated by your hamstring flexibility.

Variation: Add some power into this exercise by lowering the bar under control and exploding the weight back up to the starting position and finishing with a powerful shrug, up on your toes. You can use either a barbell or dumbbells with this exercise.

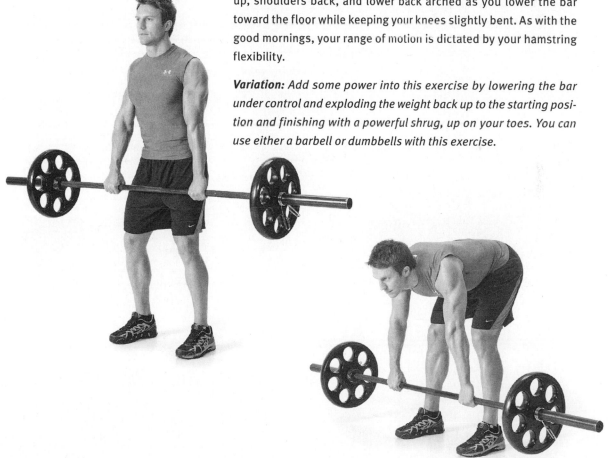

BACK EXTENSION

A common exercise seen in most gyms. This is one hip-dominant exercise where your knees are essentially fully locked out during the movement. The 45-degree-angle back-extension benches are a little easier than the standard 90-degree benches. Keep this in mind when choosing a weight to hold during the movement. You will add weight to this exercise once you can complete 10 repetitions with your body weight.

Set yourself up on the bench with your feet firmly set under the heel rests. Lower your torso into a full range of motion (make sure you are not too low on the pad so as not to limit your range). Drive upward to return to the starting position. Make sure to maintain your standard breathing pattern of inhaling at the top and exhaling as you approach the midpoint of the upward phase.

Tip: Where you place your hands can make this movement easier or harder. Arms held behind your hips is easiest, arms across the chest is moderate, and hands behind the head is the most difficult. When using a weight, hold it close to your body around the chest area.

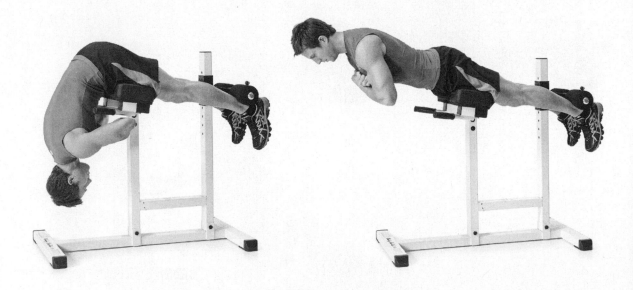

Supine Hip Extension

This is a very simple exercise and a great lead-up movement to prepare beginners for other hip-dominant exercises. This exercise has three levels of difficulty: the first is to keep your legs straight, the second is to bend your legs, and the third is to place your feet on a Swiss ball.

Lying flat on the ground, place your heels up on a bench so that your hips are on the floor and your feet are raised (legs can be straight or bent). Place your arms out on the floor to your sides. Contract your posterior chain muscles to raise your hips until they are fully extended. Pause for a count and lower back to the starting position. While your breathing pattern is not as critical in this movement as with most other exercises, try to keep the inhale to the eccentric (down) phase and the exhale on the concentric (up phase).

Tip: *Bringing your arms in closer to your body makes the movement a little more difficult due to less stability. Crossing them over your chest makes it even tougher.*

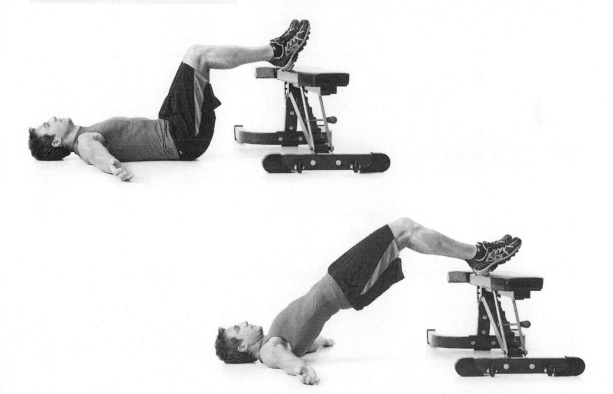

SWISS BALL
GLUTE-HAMSTRING

This is a great posterior chain exercise that is a tougher variation of the supine hip extension. The added dimensions to this exercise are twofold: One, the Swiss ball is unstable, thus requiring more strength to maintain position on the ball, and two, we are adding knee flexion of the hamstring muscle group.

Lying flat on the ground, place your heels up on a Swiss ball with your hips on the floor. As with the supine hip extension, place your arms on the floor away from your body. Contract your posterior chain muscles to raise your hips until they are fully extended. At this point you will start to perform a leg curl, flexing the knees as your heels drive into the ball and the ball moves toward your body. Pause for a count and lower back to the starting position. Follow the same breathing pattern as the supine hip extension.

Tip: *Moving your arms closer to the body increases difficulty. Crossing your arms over your chest makes this exercise quite difficult!*

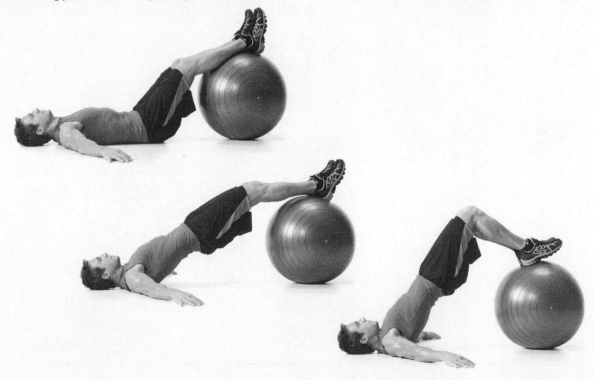

REVERSE HYPEREXTENSION

This exercise may look like a back extension, but when you perform it, the exercise will have a much different feel. This is a great change-up exercise in your routine.

Set up on a 90-degree back-extension bench facing the opposite of a standard back extension. Place your hips on the pads and hold onto the back of the bench (where your feet normally go). Either with no external load or with a medicine ball or dumbbell between your ankles, raise your legs until they are parallel with your upper body.

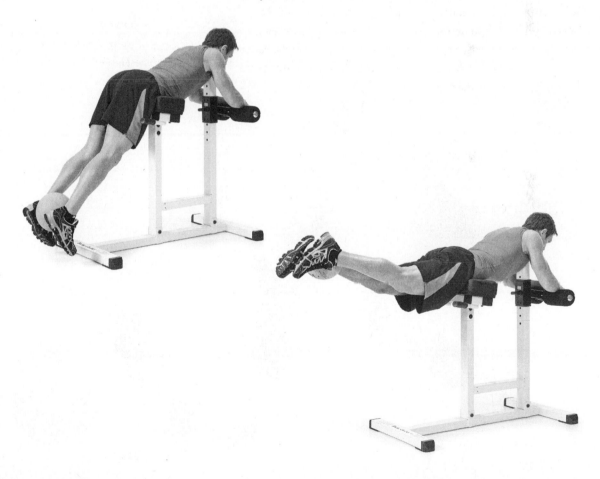

SINGLE-LEG GOOD MORNING

Just like it sounds, folks: We are talking about the same good morning exercise, but this time performing it on one leg. This is a much tougher exercise due to the balance factor.

The setup mirrors that of the standard good morning. Slightly bend one knee and pick up the other foot behind you and try to keep it off the floor for the entire set of reps. Make sure to keep the knee slightly bent and once again, push your hips backward, looking up, shoulders back and lower back arched. Complete all prescribed reps and then switch to the other leg.

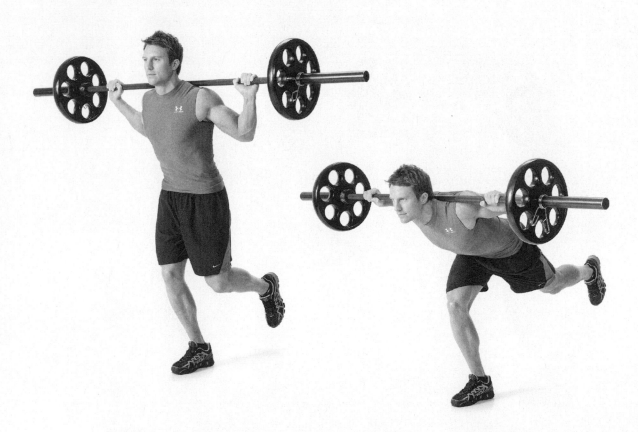

SPLIT GOOD MORNING

While this exercise is much more stable than the single-leg good morning, it places a greater load and stretch on your hamstrings due to the starting angle of the hip.

With the bar behind your neck, place one foot up on an aerobic-style step or on a couple of stacked weight plates. With your heel on the platform and toes pointed upward, keep your leg straight . Keep your back leg slightly bent. Lower down as far as possible and drive upward back to the starting position. Keep in mind that this exercise puts the hips in almost the "finished" position of a good morning (at the beginning of the exercise), so don't expect to have the same range of motion when moving downward. Complete all prescribed reps and then switch to the other leg.

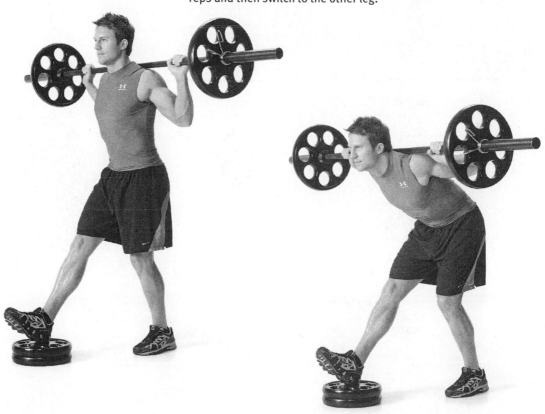

SINGLE-LEG ROMANIAN DEADLIFT

Again, this is just about identical to the standard Romanian deadlift only we are executing it on just one leg. This exercise can be performed with a barbell, two dumbbells, or one dumbbell.

Setup mirrors that of the standard Romanian deadlift. Bend your knees, picking up the other leg behind you. Try to keep it off the floor for the entire set of reps. Make sure to keep the knee slightly bent and once again, push your hips backward, looking up, shoulders back and lower back arched. Complete all prescribed reps and then switch to the other leg. When using a single dumbbell, hold it in the opposite hand of the leg that is working. Attempt to reach down and touch the dumbbell to the foot. You will raise the back leg to help counterbalance. This exercise also requires more balance.

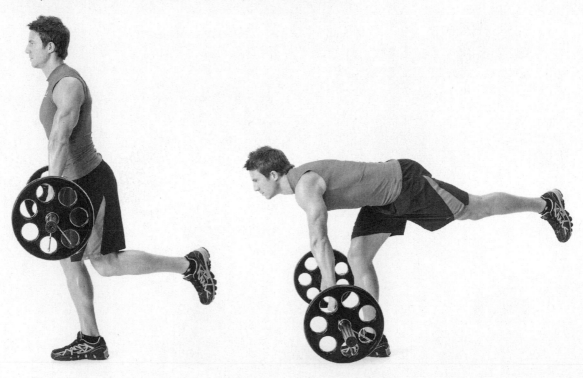

SINGLE-LEG BACK EXTENSION

While this is basically the back extension exercise, it is tougher than it looks, especially if you use a 90-degree-angle bench rather than a 45-degree-angle bench. You must attempt to contract your hamstring to try to flex your knee during the entire movement; otherwise, it will feel like a tremendous load on the extension of the knee.

Setup mirrors standard back extension. Lift one foot and place above the heel rest on the bench. Your body weight will most likely serve as adequate load for this exercise. Complete all prescribed reps with one leg and switch to the other leg.

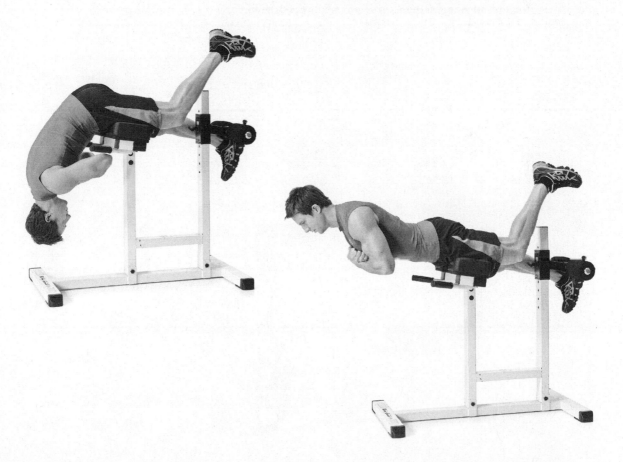

SINGLE-LEG SUPINE HIP EXTENSION

Just as the supine hip extension goes, so does the single leg. The two levels of difficulty described in the standard supine hip extension still apply with the single-leg variation.

Lying flat on the ground on your back, place your heel (leg straight) or foot (leg bent) up on a bench and hold the other leg up in the air. Contract your posterior chain muscles to raise your hips until they are fully extended. Pause for a count and lower back to the starting position. While the breathing pattern is not as critical in this movement as with most other exercises, try to keep the inhale to the eccentric (down) phase and the exhale on the concentric (up phase).

Tip: *Crossing your arms over your chest makes this single-leg variation much tougher. Complete all prescribed reps with one leg and switch to the other leg.*

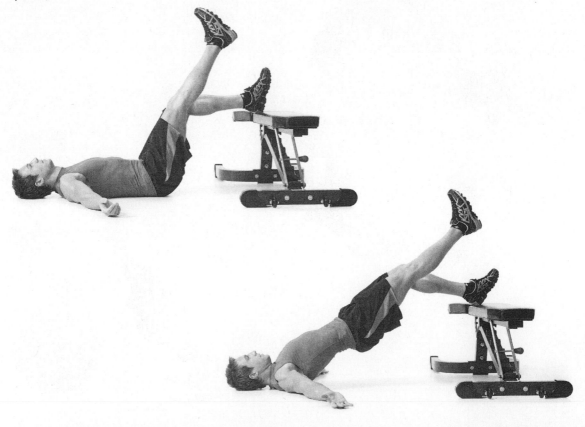

SINGLE-LEG SWISS BALL GLUTE-HAMSTRING

Okay, this is probably the most difficult of the unilaterally hip-dominant exercises, not only from a balance standpoint but from a load standpoint as well.

Lying flat on the ground on your back, place one leg (just below your calf) up on a Swiss ball, toes pointed up with hips on the floor. Hold your other leg up in the air during the movement. As with the supine hip extension, place your arms away from the body. Attempt to keep control of the ball during the entire movement, as this contributes to the difficulty.

Tip: *Only attempt the arms-crossed position when you are completely able to control the ball with ease.*

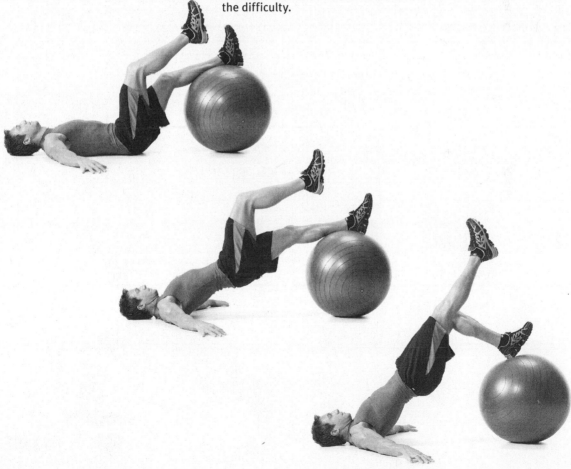

VERTICAL PUSH EXERCISES

The vertical push menu category includes all exercises that move a load vertically in the sagittal (flexion) or frontal planes of movement (abduction). This movement is usually shoulder abduction or flexion and elbow extension (in compound exercises). Picture this motion as the traditional shoulder press–style movement. I have highlighted several optional exercises in this category since this is the one menu category in which many trainees tend to experience injury issues. These options are highlighted in "Shoulder Considerations" on page 102.

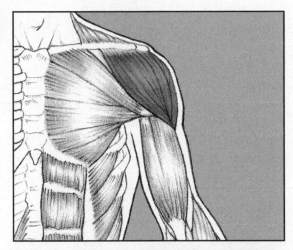

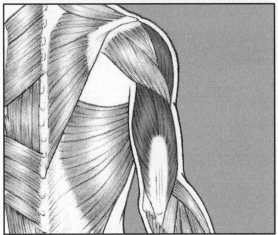

Vertical push exercises target the deltoids and the triceps (on compound movements).

97

SHOULDER PRESS

This is the most basic of all the vertical push exercises. Many of this category's exercises are just variations of the shoulder press movement. When performing any shoulder press–style exercises, be sure not to use too wide of a grip. Keep your grip at about shoulder width and think of your natural pressing motion as one that takes the bar from your shoulders past the sides of your head on the way up. Also, try to do these exercises standing rather than seated as this will increase difficulty and force your core to work as well.

Using a shoulder-width pronated grip with the bar at your shoulders (it can be placed in front of or behind the neck), press the weight up overhead. Drop your chin slightly as the bar passes your head so that it finishes above and over the head and slightly behind your ears at the top position. This is the natural movement path of your shoulders. Avoid arching backward and looking up at the weight, as this has a tendency to strain the back. Set your core at the beginning of the movement and exhale as the weight passes your head on the way up.

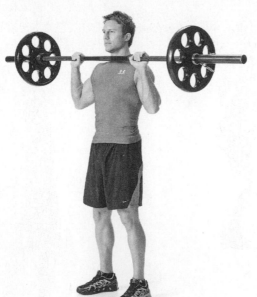
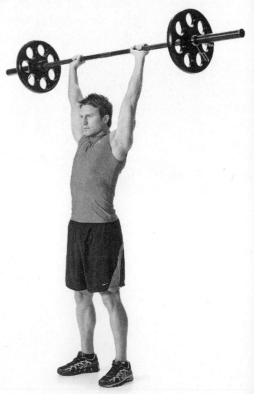

PUSH PRESS

The push press is my favorite of the vertical push exercises and one that I use quite a bit with all of my athletes. It's a great power exercise that allows you to use pretty heavy loads because your legs are involved in the movement. I like this exercise more than the traditional shoulder press as the lower body involvement allows you to drive the weight up through the "problem area" of vertical pressing exercises with less load on the shoulders.

This exercise is almost identical to the shoulder press with the exception of how the movement starts. Start with the bar either in front of or behind the neck. As you start this movement, keeping the body upright, dip downward until you are at about a quarter-squat position, and then forcefully drive upward with your legs, using this power and momentum to drive the weight overhead. Control the weight back as you lower it back down to the shoulders. You will actually shift onto your toes as you drive your legs on this movement. Your legs should be straight when the weight is locked out overhead.

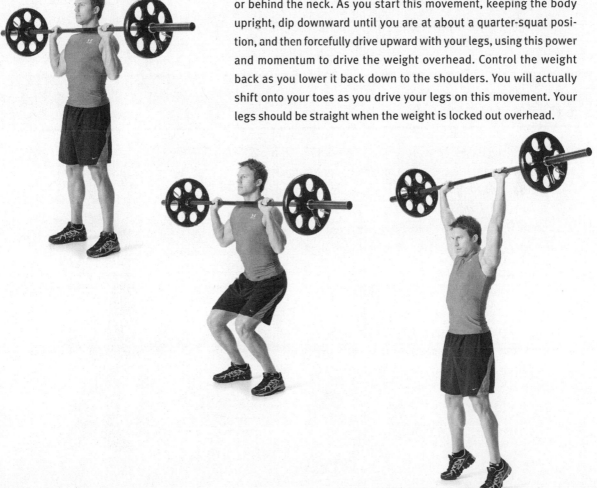

PUSH JERK

Once again, this is almost identical to the traditional shoulder press and very much like the push press because of leg involvement. The exception to this exercise is that after you drive with the legs, you will rebend your knees to get under the bar in what I call a catching base (see page 60). This base is slightly wider than your starting base with knees bent and hips back. In terms of how much load you can handle, the sequence should be shoulder press, push press, then push jerks from low to high.

Set up exactly as a push press, making sure to dip in the quarter-squat and drive with your legs. As the bar starts to reach full extension, jump the feet out slightly wider than the starting base and bend your knees to drop slightly under the bar. This is the "catch" phase of the push jerk.

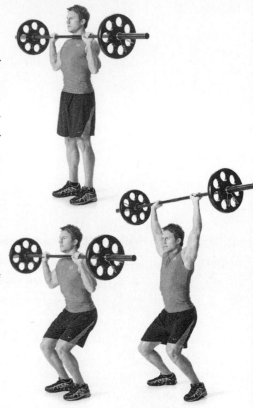

SPLIT JERK

Think of the push jerk now, but change one thing—the placement of your feet at the end of the movement or the catch phase. With the split jerk, you will catch the bar overhead with your feet split front to back rather than out to the sides. The timing cue you should watch for is the simultaneous extension of your arms and the sound of your front foot hitting the ground.

Tip: *Make sure you bring your feet back to the starting position before lowering the bar back down to your shoulders.*

Set up exactly as a push jerk, making sure to dip in the quarter-squat and drive with your legs. As the bar starts to reach full extension, jump your front foot forward and your back foot straight back. Your front leg should be bent and your back leg should act sort of like a kickstand (with a slight bend in the knee). Make sure to alternate the split leg each rep.

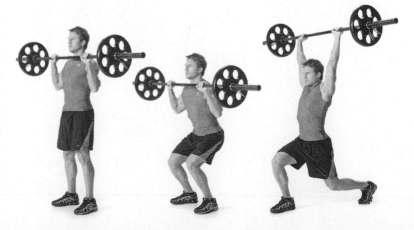

JACKKNIFE PUSHUP

Sometimes called an inverted pushup or handstand pushup, the jackknife pushup is a tremendous exercise to target your shoulders and to force your core to stabilize your body during the movement. This exercise has several levels of difficulty: the first is with feet on the floor; the next is to place your feet up on a bench (as shown); and the third is to place your feet on an unstable surface such as a Swiss ball.

Set your hands on the floor as if you were going to perform a wide-grip pushup. Now walk your feet up toward your hands so that you are in a jackknife position with your hips at the highest point and your torso almost completely inverted. Keep your head in a neutral position and lower your body until your head touches the floor, then drive up back to the starting position.

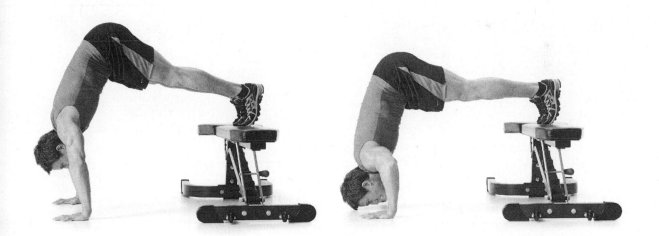

SHOULDER CONSIDERATIONS

The shoulder joint can be finicky at times. The sheer number and variety of movements this joint is capable of coupled with the fact that many people have previous injury issues often creates a potential injury time bomb. A common issue is *impingement syndrome*, in which the supraspinatus tendon of the rotator cuff is pinched against the undersurface of the acromion portion of the scapula during overhead elevation of the arm.

My friend and colleague, physical therapist Bill Hartman, sums up the potential here for injury: "Most folks are simply unprepared for overhead lifting of significant intensity due to postural issues, undesirable adaptations such as loss of motion, and isolated weaknesses. This, coupled with bad program designs and poor technique due to fatigue of the scapular stabilizers and the rotator cuff, makes impingement seem like a natural phenomenon."

If you are one of those folks who have trouble with vertical pushing exercises, here are a few exercises that can be substituted in this category.

Dumbbell Parallel-Grip Push Press

While this might still be difficult for someone with serious pressing issues, it is a more natural movement for the shoulder joint and one that's often more comfortable.

Hold dumbbells at your shoulder using a parallel grip (palms facing in). Keep your elbows forward and in front of your body. Use the push press technique to drive the weight overhead. This shoulder flexion movement should be more tolerable than the standard abduction (elbows out).

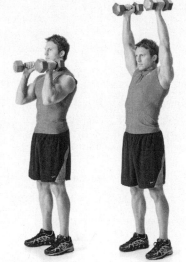

Dumbbell Scaption

This exercise targets shoulder abduction without placing the load overhead. The plane of movement also places less impingement stress on the shoulders (compared to a traditional shoulder lateral raise).

Hold dumbbells down at arm's length with palms facing forward and thumbs pointed out. Your hands should be slightly in front of your body so that the weights will travel a path about 30 degrees in front of the body (this is often called the scapular plane). Lift the dumbbells until they are even with your shoulders and then lower, keeping the weights moving in this scapular plane. The thumbs will be pointing up to the ceiling at the top of the movement.

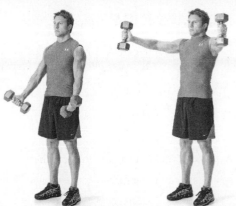

Dumbbell Scaption with Shrug

This exercise is identical to the dumbbell scaptions described above with the addition of a shrug at the top of the movement.

Plate Raise + Truck Driver

This exercise involves shoulder flexion along with internal and external rotation.

Hold a weight plate at arm's length with elbows slightly bent. Lift the weight straight out in front of your body until you can look through the hole in the weight. At this point, you will rotate the weight as far as possible (as if it were a steering wheel) both to the right and to the left and then lower the weight to the starting position. This is 1 repetition.

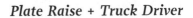
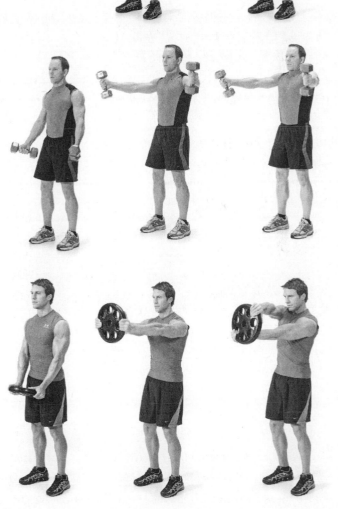

This menu category is very similar to the bilateral vertical push menu. You can make a shoulder press, push press, push jerk, and split jerk a unilateral movement simply by using dumbbells and following the same exercise techniques. By using only one dumbbell with these exercises, you can tax the core a bit more due to the uneven loading on the body. Here are a few unilateral variations that I really like. Keep in mind that most of the dumbbell exercises also can be performed with a ground based-style cable machine.

DUMBBELL ONE-ARM PRESS AND BEND

This is a great exercise for incorporating some great core work during shoulder training.

Hold one dumbbell at shoulder height with a parallel grip and place your opposite hand on your hip. Press the weight overhead and start to pronate your grip as the weight moves upward. As the weight starts to approach the full range of motion, lean your torso in the opposite direction so that the weight finishes over the opposite ear rather than directly above the shoulder.

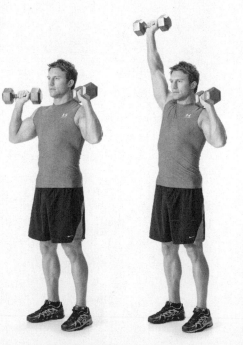

DUMBBELL ALTERNATING PRESS

Hold dumbbells at the shoulders and press one overhead. As you start to lower this weight, immediately begin pressing the opposite dumbbell. You should always have one weight moving up while the other is moving down.

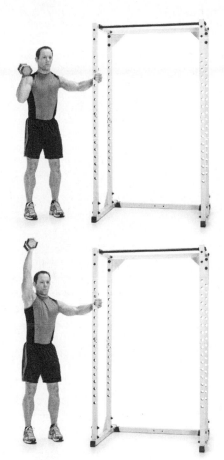

SUPPORTED DUMBBELL ONE-ARM PRESS

While exercise takes some of the core stabilization out of the equation, you will be able to handle a little more weight with this.

Hold one dumbbell at shoulder level with your opposite hand holding onto something firm (like a squat rack or other fixed machine). Press the weight overhead.

SIDE-TO-SIDE JACKKNIFE PUSHUP

This is performed the same as the jackknife pushups described earlier with the difference being that you will lower yourself toward one shoulder as you descend before pushing back to the start and repeating to the other shoulder. Turning your head slightly toward the shoulder will help with this movement.

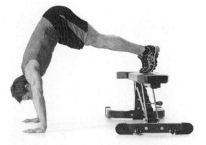
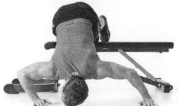
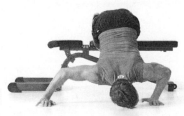

VERTICAL PULL EXERCISES

The vertical pull menu category includes all exercises that move a load vertically in the sagittal (extension), frontal, or transverse planes (adduction). The exercises in this category involve shoulder extension or adduction with elbow flexion (on compound exercises). Picture these motions as the traditional pullup or close-grip seated row movements.

While I mentioned in the last chapter that the shoulder joint is one that often experiences problems with overhead pushing movements, the same is not as common with vertical pulling exercises. As Bill Hartman would explain it, "The compression loads (vertical push) are far more wearing on the shoulder joint than the traction loads found during vertical or horizontal pulling exercises." Therefore, someone who has previous shoulder injury issues might actually have no problems performing any or all of the vertical pull menu exercises.

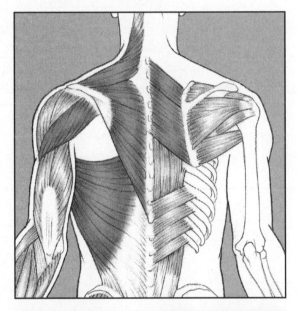

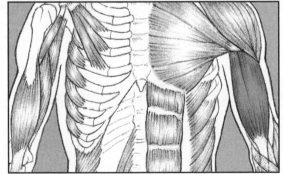

Vertical pull exercises target the latissimus dorsi, rear deltoids, trapezius, rhomboids, and biceps.

CHINUP

The chinup is probably the most well known and one of the most effective of all the vertical pull exercises. Whether you need assistance to complete them or not, chinups are one exercise that should be included in your training. As with all of the vertical pulling exercises, make sure to get a full range of motion when performing these movements. In other words, start the exercises with your arms completely extended and finish with a complete pull.

Tip: *Use an assisted chinup machine, a heavy-duty rubber band, or even a bench under your feet for assistance if you are unable to complete the prescribed number of repetitions.*

Using a supinated grip (palms facing your body) with your hands narrower than shoulder width, start in a complete hanging position under a fixed bar. Drive your elbows down and back to raise your body until your chin is above the bar. Chinups target shoulder extension on the sagittal plane.

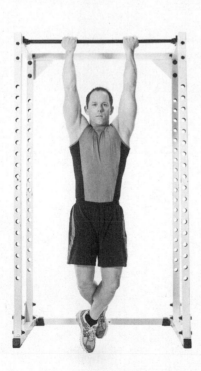
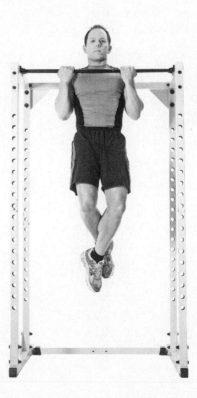

PULLUP

Tip: *Use assistance if necessary to complete all of the prescribed repetitions.*

Pullups tend to be a bit more difficult than chinups but are essentially very similar. I recommend either alternating between chinups and pullups during workouts or at least alternating them from workout to workout to assure that the shoulder joint is being trained on both sagittal and frontal planes.

Using a pronated grip (palms facing away from you) with hands slightly wider than shoulder width, start in a complete hanging position under a fixed bar. Drive your elbows out and down to raise your body until your chin is above the bar. Pullups target shoulder adduction on the frontal plane.

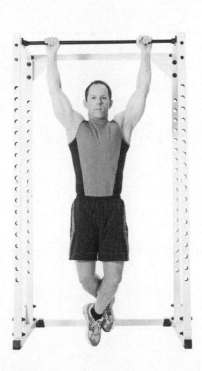 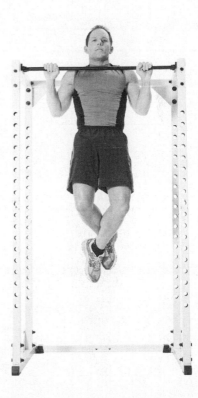

MIXED-GRIP PULLUP

This is one of my favorite pullup variations and one that essentially involves both the pullup and chinup mechanics simultaneously.

Using a mixed grip (one hand supinated and the other pronated) with your hands no wider than shoulder width, start in a complete hanging position under a fixed bar. To pull your body up you will actually have the supinated arm doing chinup mechanics (elbow in) and the pronated arm doing pullup mechanics (elbow out) to get your chin over the bar. Once again, use assistance if needed. Make sure to change grips on each set so that you are not always using the same mix.

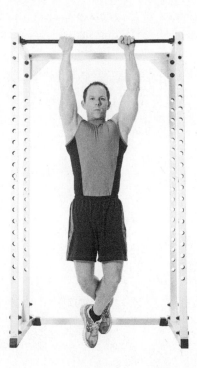
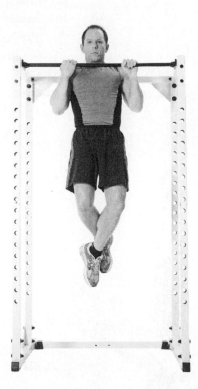

LAT PULLDOWN

This is usually the exercise you see folks doing when they aren't very good at pullups, right? Well, this is a solid exercise that allows you to get your vertical pulling volume in when you don't have access to a pullup bar or are unable to find a way to self-spot. As with the pullup variations, make sure to use a full range of motion and avoid leaning back too far as you pull the weight down. We have all seen the guy pulling the bar down to his belly on this exercise, right? Well, don't do this. Bring the bar down to just the upper chest, as this will complete the range of motion requirements.

You have your choice of grips when doing lat pulldowns. Just keep in mind that, as with pullups, different grips tend to incorporate different shoulder muscles. When using a wider, pronated grip, you will be targeting shoulder adduction on the frontal plane. When using a closer, supinated grip, you will be targeting shoulder extension on the sagittal plane. Like the pullups, I recommend alternating between sets or at least workout to workout.

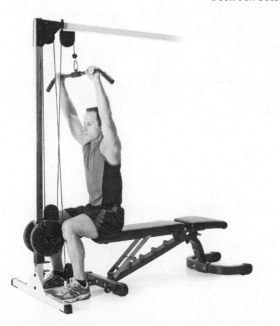 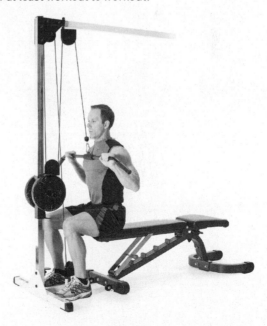

POWER TRAINING SHOULDER REHAB TIPS

If using a pronated or supinated grip on pullup or lat-pulldown variations tends to irritate your shoulders, don't give up! Try a parallel grip, in which the hands face inward toward the body with thumbs facing backward. Most gyms have a pulldown attachment and a pullup bar fixture to facilitate this grip. This grip tends to place less stress on the shoulders due to less internal and external rotation during the movement. Also, try leaning back to about a 30-degree angle during your pulldowns, as this will also alleviate potential impingement issues.

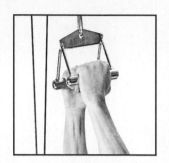

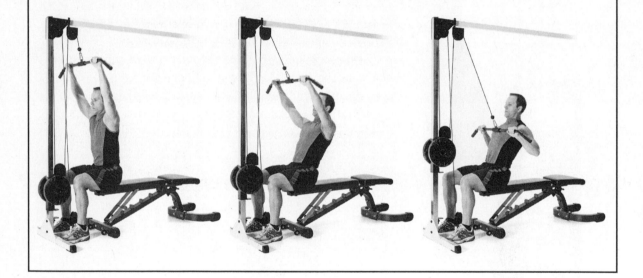

SINGLE-ARM PULLDOWN OR PULLUP

Okay, while a single-arm lat pulldown won't prove to be difficult, almost everybody will need significant assistance when trying to do single-arm pullup variations. This is where assistance machines come in handy. As with the bilateral vertical pull exercises already mentioned, try to alternate between elbow in and elbow out while executing the pulling motions.

PULLDOWN

Use a single-handle attachment and set up just as you would a regular lat pulldown. Maintain an erect torso and try not to lean one way or the other during the pulldown. Pull down until the handle is even with your shoulder.

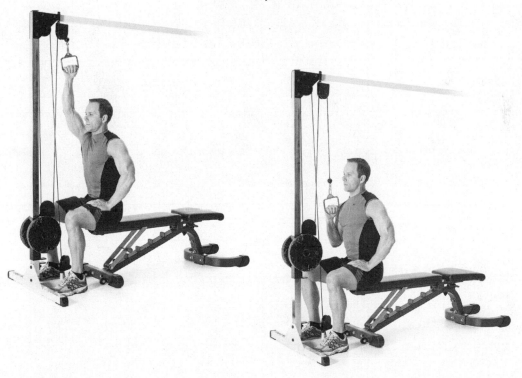

PULLUP

Use either an assisted pullup machine, a heavy-duty rubber band, or a spotter, and perform the same range of motion as a traditional pullup or chinup.

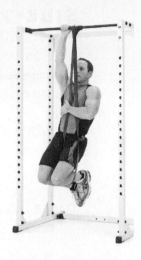
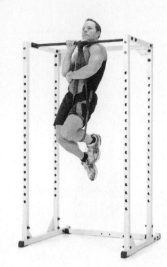

PULLUPS TOO EASY?

While this is not usually a problem, some individuals will occasionally be able to do more than the prescribed amount of repetitions. If this is the case, you must create overload by adding weight to the movement.

My favorite way to add weight on any exercise is to wear a weighted vest. Vests are great because they do not cause any discomfort as compared to weighted belts. A weighted belt is the next best option and a better option if you need to add a significant amount of weight to your exercise since vests generally come in 10- to 20-pound ranges.

You can find these bands and vests from Perform Better at www.performbetter.com.

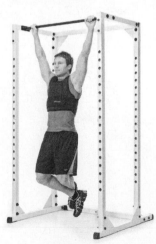
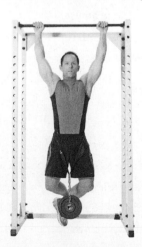
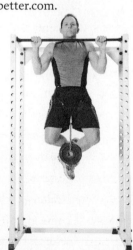

SIDE-TO-SIDE PULLUP

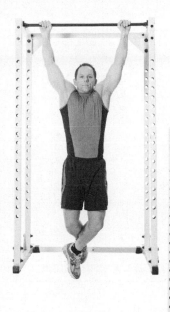

While this is still technically a bilateral movement, the shifting of the weight during the exercise will place greater load on one limb. Give this exercise a try; I think you'll really get a kick out of it!

Use a pronated grip, slightly wider than your pullup grip. From a hanging position, pull yourself up and toward one of your hands until your chin touches the back of your hand. Lower and repeat to the other side. Each lift is 1 repetition. *Note:* This side-to-side technique is not as effective when using a lat pull-down cable.

CAN'T DO A SINGLE PULLUP?

Well, don't worry. A product called the Jump Stretch FlexBand has emerged in the conditioning world. This is an extra strong rubber band that is used to assist during body-weight exercises like pullups, dips, and so forth. It's a great tool for those who can't perform pullup variations on their own, can only complete a few repetitions, or just need a way to self-spot during training.

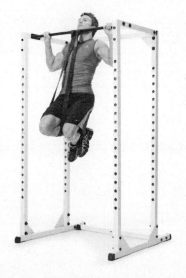

I have used these super bands extensively with many of my athletes and have seen amazing improvements in pullup performance. In fact, I have had individuals who started out not being able to complete a single pullup, and after a 12-week training cycle, could complete 3 to 5 on their own.

The bands come in different widths so you can graduate to a smaller and smaller one until you are doing them on your own.

HORIZONTAL PUSH EXERCISES

The horizontal push menu category includes all the exercises that move a load horizontally in the sagittal (shoulder flexion) or transverse planes of movement (shoulder adduction). In addition to the movement at the shoulder, you will also be extending your elbow to include the triceps. A typical example of this type of movement is a traditional bench press with elbows out (transverse) or a close-grip bench press with elbows in (sagittal). The menu of exercises is pretty basic, but there are many exercise variations that allow you to vary your training quite a bit. Feel free to mix up your grips from regular to close grip to reverse grip (see "Bar Grip Variations" on page 121) each time you train using the horizontal push menu.

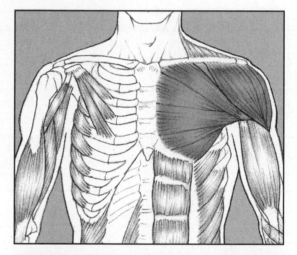

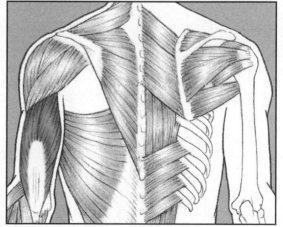

Horizontal push exercises target the pectorals, anterior deltoids, and triceps.

BENCH PRESS

The bench press is easily the most popular resistance training exercise on the planet. This is the one exercise that rarely requires an introduction because most everybody knows how to do it.

On a flat bench, using a slightly wider-than-shoulder-width grip, lower the bar to the center of your chest. Drive the bar upward and slightly backward (toward the head) until your arms are fully extended. Unless you have an injury, I recommend completing a *full* range of motion on this and all exercises. On the bench press movements, this means bringing the bar down until it touches your chest and extending your elbows completely at the end of the lift.

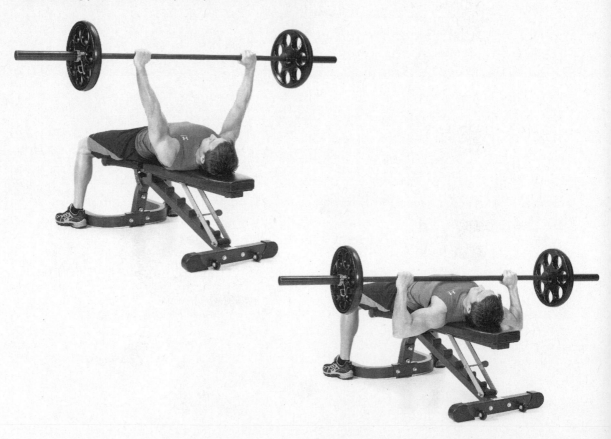

INCLINE BENCH PRESS

While it is more or less a matter of personal preference, the angle of the incline is generally set at about 30 to 45 degrees. Keep in mind that the greater the angle, the weaker the movement gets. Also, the greater the angle, the greater the stress on the shoulders. Therefore, you want to find the optimal angle that still allows you to primarily train the chest.

Perform the same movements as the flat bench press, only lower the weight to a spot higher up on the chest toward your collarbone.

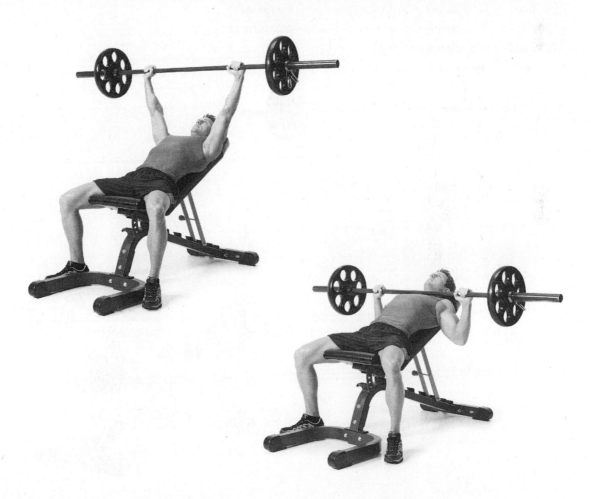

CLOSE-GRIP BENCH PRESS

As I mentioned in the introduction of the menu categories, it is important to address the push and pull exercises on all the planes through which the body will move through during exercises. By moving your grip in closer and keeping your elbows in, we can target shoulder flexion in the sagittal plane rather than shoulder adduction in the transverse plane. A marker I use to measure the close grip is extending your thumbs and touching the ends together; this is approximately your close grip.

Perform the same movements as the regular bench press, only now you will attempt to keep your elbows tight to your body as you lower and raise the weight. Due to the change in the shoulder movement, the location of where the bar touches the chest will also be slightly lower than the regular bench press.

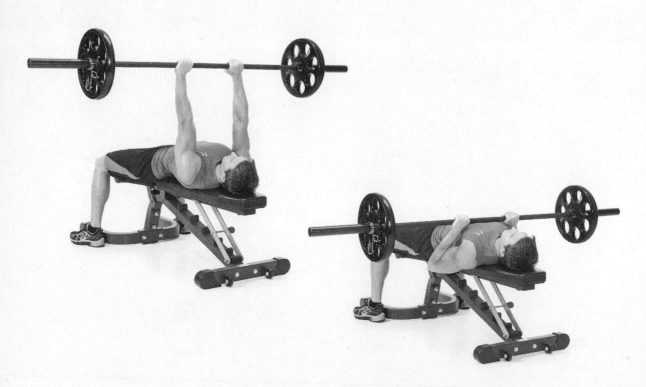

CLOSE-GRIP INCLINE PRESS

This is one of my favorite horizontal push exercises, as it is very tough and a great strength builder.

As with the regular incline, set the angle to your personal preference. Keep your elbows tight to the body as you lower and raise the weight. The contact point on your chest will now be around the nipple line.

BAR GRIP VARIATIONS

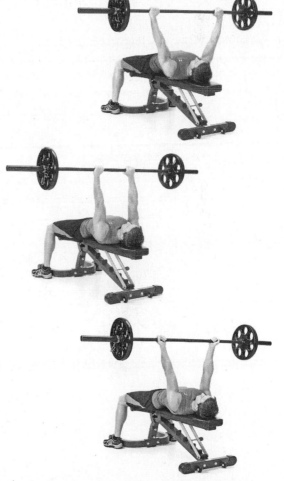

Regular Grip

Overhand, slightly wider than shoulder width.

Close Grip

Overhand, hands approximately 10 inches apart, elbows in.

Reverse Grip

Underhand, hands slightly wider than shoulder width, elbows in. This grip is much like the close grip, as the elbows are forced in during the movement.

REVERSE-GRIP BENCH PRESS

This is similar to the traditional bench press, only you're using a supinated grip. This exercise targets the anterior deltoids and triceps a bit more.

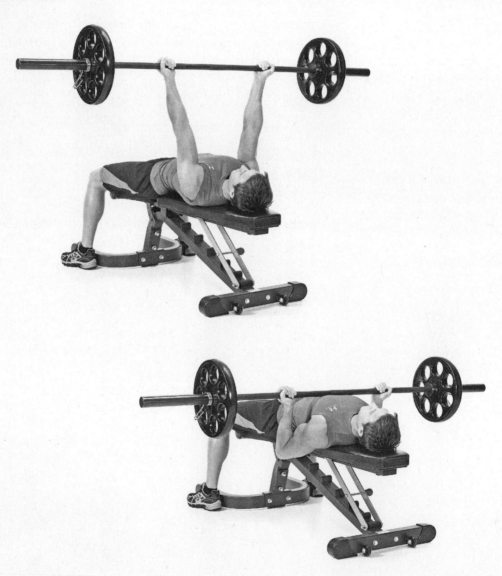

PUSHUPS

Pushups are a great exercise in the horizontal push category. What I love most about pushups is the fact that, unlike doing a bench press on a bench, the core must play its role in supporting the body. Otherwise, you will inevitably fail in performing this exercise due to improper form. The drawback in choosing push-ups from this category is that you may be strong enough to do more repetitions than prescribed in the program. In this case, you could still do pushup variations; you would just need an external load (i.e., weighted vest, partner, elevate your feet, etc.) to make the exercise tougher. I will go through the pushup variations below.

FLAT PUSHUP

Tip: *Moving your hands closer together will make the exercise more difficult, as this places greater stress on the shoulders and triceps.*

Hands should be slightly wider than shoulder-width apart. Keeping your abs tight and back flat, lower until your chest touches the floor. Drive up until your arms are completely extended.

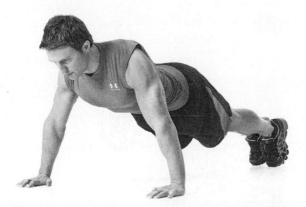

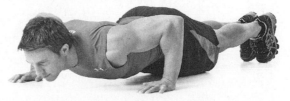

DECLINE PUSHUP

Performed the same way as a regular flat pushup except on a bench or a chair, this exercise is easier as the angle creates less load on the body.

Tip: Doing these on a Swiss ball will make the exercise more difficult due to the added instability, requiring more work from your core.

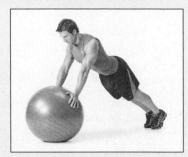

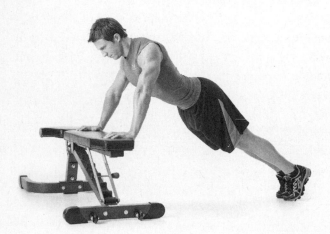

INCLINE PUSHUP

Performed like a regular pushups, only now you will be increasing the load by raising your feet onto a bench or chair. Focus on stabilizing your core as the hips have a tendency to sink during this exercise.

Tip: Placing your feet on a Swiss ball will make this exercise much more difficult due to increased instability, making it a great core movement.

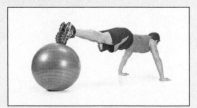

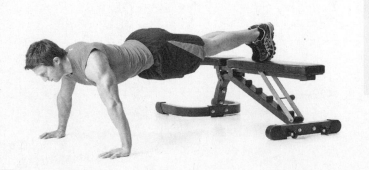

DIP

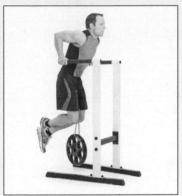

This is a great exercise in this category because much like chinups and pullups, dips force you to handle your body weight in a difficult, more unsupported situation.

Using a grip slightly wider than the width of your body, lower your body until your upper arms are at least parallel to the ground. Try to keep your torso erect with only a slight lean forward. Drive up until your arms are fully extended. I will caution you against something I often see in the gym: Many people have a tendency to use too wide of a grip when performing dips, thus placing their shoulders at a greater risk for injury. Try to keep your grip slightly outside the width of your body.

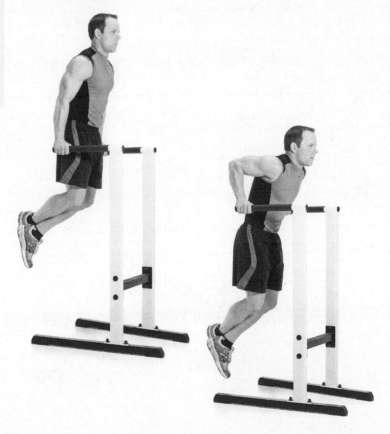

DUMBBELL BENCH PRESSES

This is the simplest way to transform a traditional exercise from a bilateral to a unilateral. By using dumbbells instead of a bar, you will force your limbs to work independently and promote strength and muscular balance. Keep in mind that because of this new instability and limb independence, the loads will feel heavier. In other words, if you can bench-press 300 pounds for a 1-rep maximum, you will not be able to perform a 1-rep maximum with 150-pound dumbbells. Let's review some of the variations.

NOTES ON DUMBBELL POSITIONING

Getting the Dumbbells in Place

In a seated position, place the dumbbells on your thighs. Using your legs to help, push the weights up to your shoulders as you lower yourself back onto the bench.

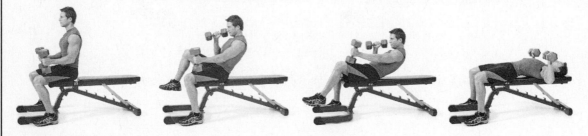

Getting the Dumbbells Back to the Seated Position

With your arms extended and the dumbbells over your chest, bring your feet up so that your hips are at a 90-degree angle. Bring the dumbbells to your thighs and push yourself back up to the seated position using the momentum of the weight.

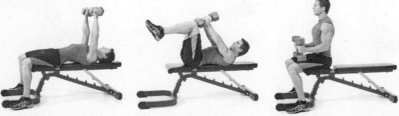

DUMBBELL FLAT BENCH OR INCLINE BENCH PRESS

Using the procedures mentioned earlier to place the dumbbells in starting position, perform a bench press by evenly lowering the weights until they are even with (touch) your outer chest. Drive the weights up until your arms are fully extended.

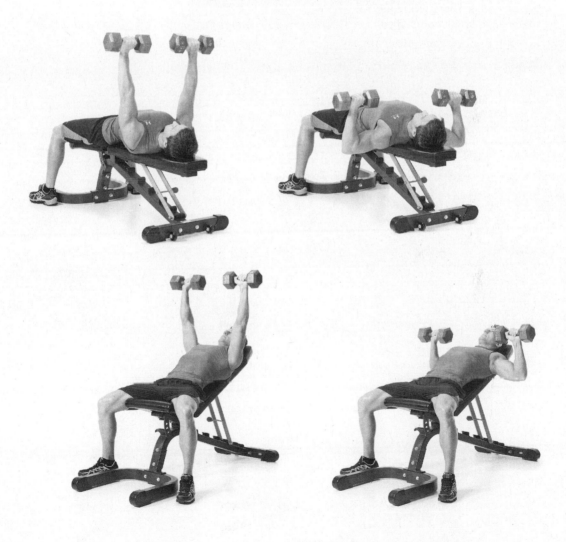

DUMBBELL ALTERNATING BENCH PRESS

As with the regular dumbbell bench press, get yourself into position. Lower one dumbbell to the bottom position and then drive it upward. As you are driving the dumbbell upward, simultaneously lower the other dumbbell. The movement should resemble two pistons, as both will be constantly moving.

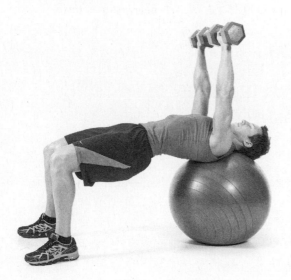

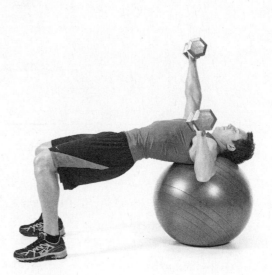

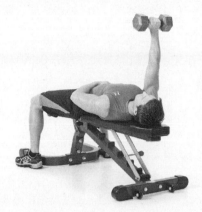

ONE-ARM DUMBBELL FLAT BENCH OR INCLINE BENCH PRESS

This can be a much more difficult exercise due to increased instability. When using two dumbbells, the loads counterbalance themselves. Using one dumbbell, you will encounter a shift in load and will have to use the rest of your body to keep the load balanced. With one dumbbell, perform a flat or incline bench press while keeping the other arm either out to the side or across your torso.

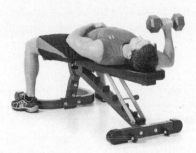

DUMBBELL TRAINING TIPS

Using dumbbells allows you to change your grip from an overhand to a parallel, or neutral, grip. When using a parallel grip, you are performing the shoulder flexion movement on the sagittal plane. This grip is also easier on the shoulders for those with injury issues during horizontal press movements.

Using a Swiss ball instead of a bench can add difficulty to any of the dumbbell exercises described in this book. When using a ball for the flat bench variations, make sure that your head and shoulders are firmly supported on the ball and your hips are held high with your torso stable. When using a ball for an incline variation, simply drop your hips down so that you create an adequate incline angle to perform your exercises. The single-arm press movements are especially challenging when using a Swiss ball.

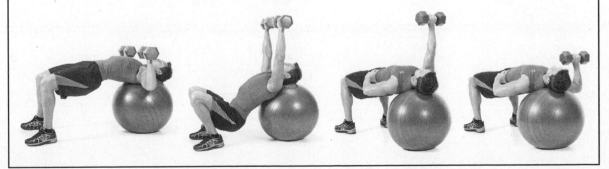

SIDE-TO-SIDE PUSHUP

As with the regular pushups, these can be done from a flat, incline, or decline position.

Using a hand placement slightly wider than your regular pushup width, descend toward the floor by moving toward one hand. Your body will shift completely to that side. Push back up to the starting position and repeat the movement to the other side. While you are still using both limbs to push, you are significantly placing greater load on one side at a time.

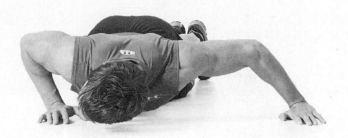

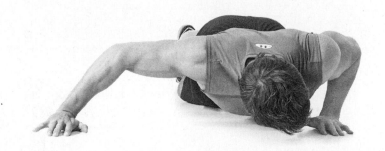

STANDING CABLE CHEST PRESS

This is a tremendous functional exercise because it addresses the horizontal push from a standing, unsupported position. These can be done with one or both arms at the same time (if you have a two-cable pulley system).

Stand with a stable base of support with feet either even or slightly staggered. Starting with the cable handle even with your chest, drive the load as if you are punching at something.

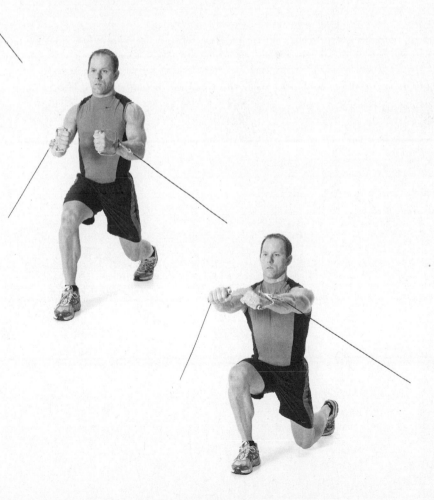

HORIZONTAL PULL EXERCISES

This horizontal pull menu category includes all the exercises that move a load horizontally in the sagittal (extension) or transverse planes of movement (abduction). In addition to the movement at the shoulder, there will also be a flexion of the elbow tying in biceps movement. Typical examples of this type of movement are (A) cable row with elbows in (sagittal) or (B) cable row to the neck with elbows out (transverse).

As with the horizontal pushing exercises, the simple shift of movement from a close grip with elbows in close to the body to a wide grip with elbows out will change the movement planes of all of the exercises.

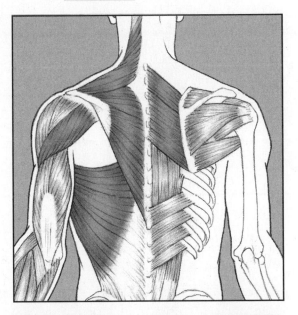

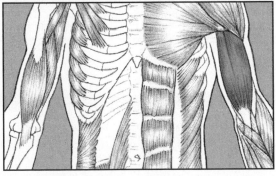

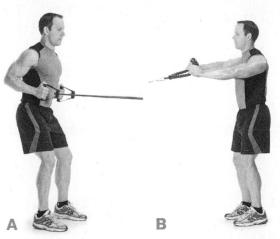

A   **B**

Horizontal pull exercises target the latissimus dorsi, rear deltoids, rhomboids, trapezius, and biceps.

BENT-OVER ROW

This is a very common exercise but one that can be made more difficult and functional by decreasing the support. Rather than resting on a support pad during this exercise, use a regular barbell and support the load with your posterior chain and core muscles.

Start with your feet shoulder-width apart with hands slightly wider than shoulder width and hands pronated (overhand grip). Lower your torso so that you create at least a 45-degree angle at the hips. Your knees should be bent slightly and your lower back should be flat. Try to maintain a rigid torso as you move the weight. Row the weight up until the bar makes contact with the lower rib cage. Lower the bar until your arms are completely extended.

Tip: *Try supinating your hands (underhand grip) and using a close grip to target the sagittal plane movement of the row.*

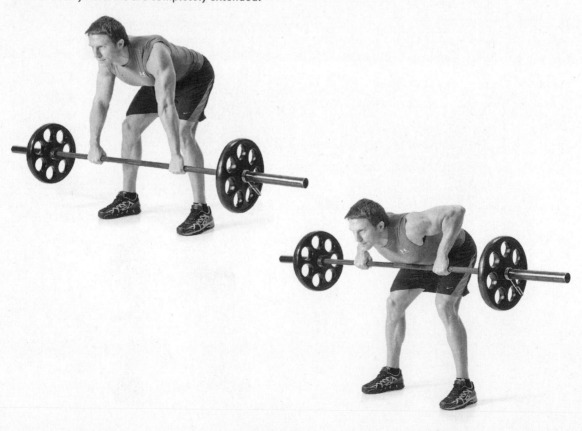

MODIFIED T-BAR ROW

Traditionally, this exercise is done using a bar with a "T" handle while placing your chest on a support pad. Use a regular Olympic bar held with hands together.

Tip: *Lean slightly backward as you pull the weight to make sure the bar is pivoting at the corner during the exercise.*

Place one end of an Olympic bar in a wall corner (use a towel to cover the end that is in contact with the corner to avoid damaging the wall and the bar). Place weights on the other bar end. Straddling the bar and facing away from the corner, grip the bar with both hands in a double closed-fist fashion close to the weights. Keep your body in the same position as the bent-over row and perform the rows while straddling the bar, making sure to complete a full range of motion.

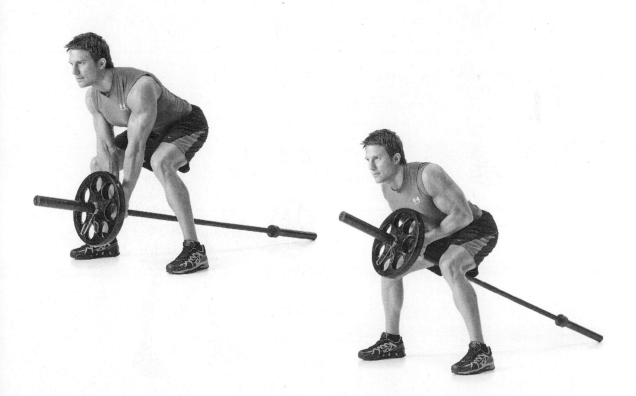

HORIZONTAL PULLUP

A tremendous exercise that allows you to handle your body weight in much the same way as in a traditional pullup. This exercise has three levels of difficulty: feet on the floor (shown on the opposite page), feet on a bench (shown below), and feet on a Swiss ball (shown below). In addition, the lower the bar placement, the more difficult the exercise.

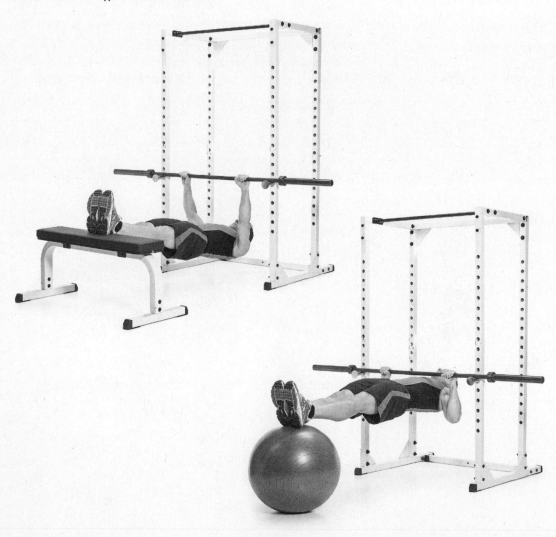

Tip: *As the reps become more difficult to complete, bend your knees slightly and bring the feet a bit closer to the bar. This makes the movement easier. Also, remember to regularly change your grips from wide with elbows out to narrow with elbows in. You can even supinate (palms up) your grip when doing the narrow pulls.*

Set a standard Olympic bar on a squat rack so it is high enough to hang underneath without your back touching the floor. If this position is too difficult, raise the bar. You can also use a Smith machine. Hang underneath the bar with legs extended and your body stiff and tight. Pull up until your chest almost touches the bar (slightly above the nipple line) and lower until your arms are completely extended.

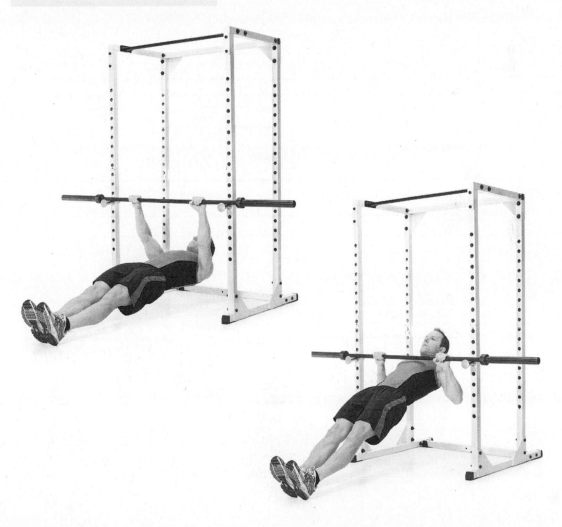

STANDING CABLE ROW TO RIB CAGE

This exercise changes the angles of the horizontal pull and allows you to perform a traditional seated cable row from a standing, unsupported position.

Use a narrow grip handle or a close grip on a straight handle. With feet shoulder-width apart, knees slightly bent, and abs tight, pull the weight toward you until the handle contacts your lower rib cage. Extend the weight back out until your arms are completely extended.

Tip: *If possible, alternate from performing this exercise with the cable starting from a low position to a waist-high position.*

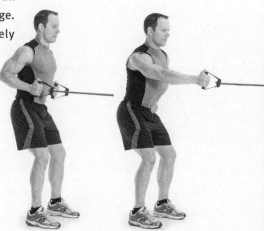

REHAB CORNER: SHOULDER CONSIDERATIONS

My friend and colleague, Bill Hartman, has described an exercise called the face pull as one of the most underrated horizontal pulling exercises. The position of the hands and the movement at the shoulder helps develop important scapular stabilization, which is often lacking in people with shoulder issues. Take a look at this great exercise.

Cable Face Pull

This is performed like a traditional cable row only using a rope attachment. Vary the position of the cable from low, to level, to high from workout to workout. Holding the rope attachment with a neutral grip (thumbs up), row the weight upward toward your ears.

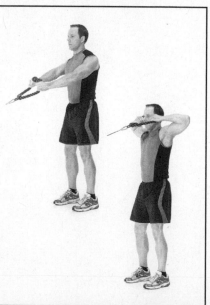

STANDING CABLE ROW TO NECK

This exercise is also performed from the standing position, but now you will be pulling the load to your neck with your elbows out. This emphasizes the transverse plane movement of the pull and also places greater stress on the rear deltoids.

Use a rope handle to allow the hands to come apart naturally at the end of the movement. If you do not have one, use a standard straight bar with somewhat of a closer grip (thumbs in, elbows out). To perform this exercise, start with the pulley aligned at waist height. If you start too low, you will consequently perform an upright row, which is not what you should be aiming for here.

If you only have a low pulley system, then move to a seated position for this exercise. As you pull the weight toward your neck, drive your elbows out and back as if you're squeezing your shoulder blades together at the top. Return the weight by fully extending your arms to the starting position.

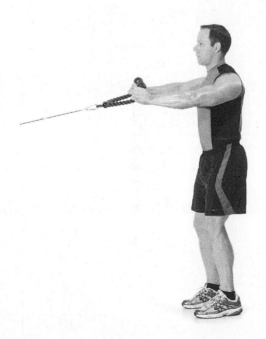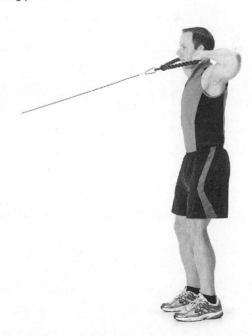

BENT-OVER DUMBBELL ALTERNATING ROW

This movement is essentially the direct opposite of the dumbbell alternating horizontal press in the last chapter. It's a great exercise that requires lots of core stabilization due to the constant movement.

Start with feet shoulder-width apart and torso bent forward to at least a 45-degree angle at the hips. Holding the dumbbells either with a parallel grip (palms facing in with elbows in) or a pronated grip (thumbs in and elbows out), row one dumbbell up to the rib cage and then lower it to the starting position. As the dumbbell is being lowered, the other one should start ascending. This should resemble a piston-like action, as both dumbbells will always be moving simultaneously.

Tip: Change the grips occasionally from parallel to pronated to make sure you address both planes of movement.

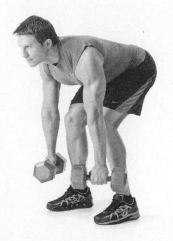 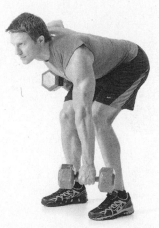 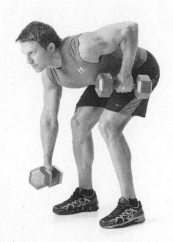

BENT-OVER TWO-POINT DUMBBELL ROW

This is a unique exercise, as you will be placed in a difficult support position. Traditionally, this exercise is performed using a bench to support the body; however, here you will rely on your body for support.

Tip: *Due to the shifting of the body, there is a tendency to perform this exercise in a higher position than the other rowing exercises. Remember to maintain an appropriate torso position with your knees bent, torso leaning forward at least 45 degrees, and lower back flat.*

Start with feet shoulder-width apart and torso bent forward to at least a 45-degree angle at the hips. When rowing with your left arm (as shown), slightly stagger your left foot back a bit to facilitate a natural rowing path for the dumbbell, and place your other hand behind your back. There will be a large shift in the load due to the weight of the dumbbell. Attempt to maintain an even position (not tilted) during the entire movement. Start by holding the dumbbell in the center of the body, row the weight up to your rib cage and then back down to the start. Repeat the reps with your other arm.

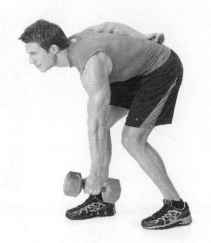 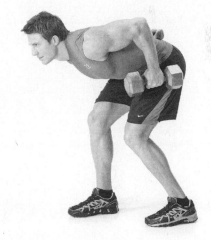

TWO-POINT DUMBBELL ROW WITH TWIST

Stand holding a dumbbell in your left hand with your left foot staggered slightly behind the right. Bench down into a good row position and place your right arm behind your back. Row the dumbbell up and rotate the shoulders as far as possible, as if you are trying to drive your elbow up and across to the right side of your body. Repeat the set on the other side.

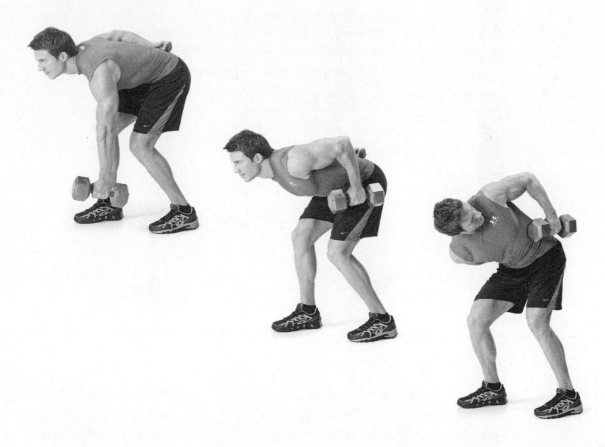

Tip: Change your movements occasionally by rowing to the rib cage and also rowing with elbows out, and bringing your hand toward your neck.

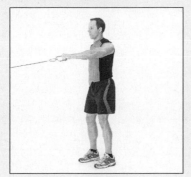

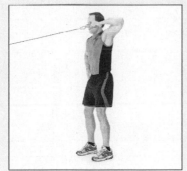

ONE-ARM STANDING CABLE ROW

This exercise is the same as the standing cable rows already described, only use one arm at a time.

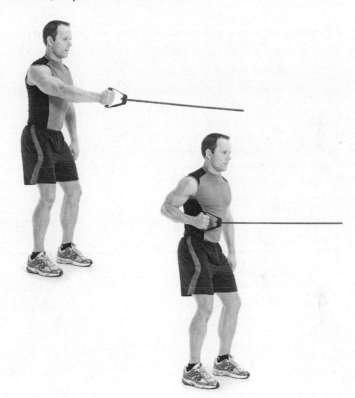

FUNCTIONAL TIP

As I have talked about numerous times throughout this book, the gold standard for most exercises is to perform them in a standing position. The same holds true for a common seated exercise, the cable row. Moving from a seated to a standing position forces your core to work to stabilize your body. As a result, the load will feel heavier from a standing position. From a standing position, this is essentially a full-body exercise. This is about as good of a functional exercise example as there is.

HORIZONTAL SIDE-TO-SIDE PULLUP

Another favorite of mine, this movement is much like the side-to-side pullup. It allows us to change a bilateral exercise to become more like a unilateral one.

Set up for a regular horizontal pullup. As you start from the hanging position, pull yourself up and toward one hand. Try to touch your chest on the back of that hand. Return to the starting position and pull to the other side on the next repetition.

Tip: Moving your hands wider apart makes this exercise more difficult. Remember that you still have the difficulty options with this exercise (floor, bench, ball) as mentioned earlier.

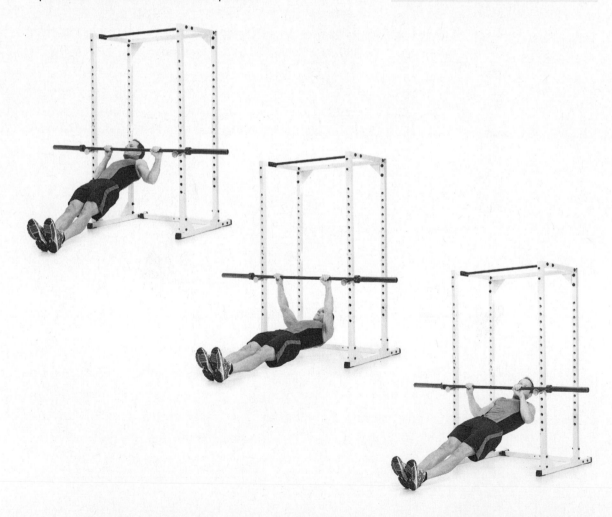

ONE-ARM HORIZONTAL PULLUP

While 99.9 percent of us out there cannot perform a one-arm pullup, many of us can, in fact, perform a one-arm horizontal pullup. This is a great body-weight exercise and a perfect option for those who don't find the regular horizontal pullup very difficult.

Set up for a regular horizontal pullup. Grab the bar with one arm, centering it with your body. Bend your knees a little bit and bring your feet in a little closer than normal. As you pull up toward the bar, reach the other arm up toward the ceiling (as if you are punching upward). Repeat the reps with the other arm.

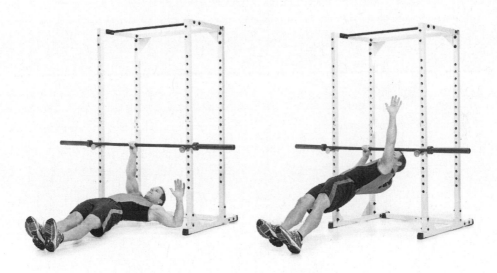

ROTATIONAL CORE EXERCISES

The *core* consists of the muscle groups that run up, down, and around the torso from the rib cage to the hips. These muscles often work in unison to perform everyday tasks such as bending, lifting, twisting. To become a strong squatter (especially a front squatter), you must have a powerful core. Even movements like standing presses and bent-over rows require substantial core strength to stabilize during these exercises (especially if the loads are heavy).

We will focus on rotational movements that work both on a parallel plane and a diagonal plane. Training rotational movements diagonally allows you to move in multiple planes; it also allows you to incorporate the rectus abdominiss and spinal erectors to work in unison as the torso flexes and extends as it rotates. This is an extremely functional movement as it mimics many everyday activities that recruit this muscle group. Essentially, we are trying to attack the entire torso region. Depending on your goals, there are times when you may want to train in a slower, more controlled fashion and other times when we may want to create as much power as possible, moving as fast as we can. For example, when you are trying to develop power, you will want to move the loads in an explosive fashion. When you are trying to develop strength and stability, you will want to move in a slower, more controlled manner. Both styles are recommended during training.

Included are strength and power exercises along with what I call *uninhibited* exercises with medicine balls that accelerate a load without decelerating it. An example would be throwing a medicine ball against a wall as hard as possible. This is impossible to replicate in a weight room with weights.

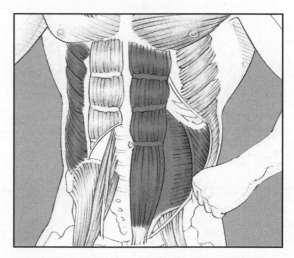

Rotational core exercises target the rectus abdominis, internal and external obliques, transverse abdominis, and spinal erectors in the back.

SEATED RUSSIAN TWIST

This is a common exercise seen in the gym, but often performed incorrectly. The most common mistake when performing this exercise is with the torso in a seated vertical or even standing position. In these positions, there is little demand on your core rotators as the load is determined by gravity. So in a vertical position, there would be little to no rotational load; the load would be vertical rather than rotational.

Tip: *The farther out you hold the weight, the tougher the exercise. With this in mind, as the set becomes too difficult, start to bend your arms more to bring the weight closer to the body.*

Start seated on the floor with your knees bent and heels in contact with the ground. Lean back until you feel the abdominals engage to stabilize your body. Holding a medicine ball or a weight plate, rotate as far as possible to your right and touch the ball or plate to the ground behind you. Make sure you rotate your entire torso and are not just reaching around with your arms. Wherever the weight goes, your shoulders and eyes should go as well. After touching, forcefully change direction and move the load to the other side (without pausing). I like to try to move the load as fast as possible in this exercise but keep in mind that the heavier the load, the slower you will actually be moving.

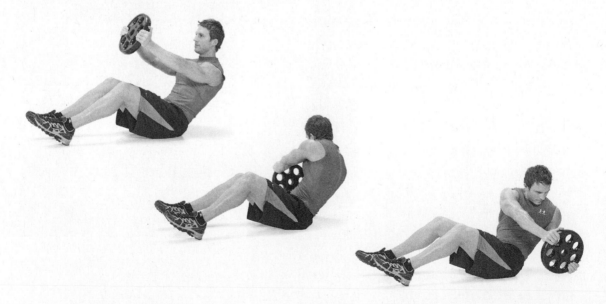

CORKSCREW

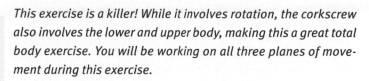

This exercise is a killer! While it involves rotation, the corkscrew also involves the lower and upper body, making this a great total body exercise. You will be working on all three planes of movement during this exercise.

Stand with feet shoulder-width apart holding a dumbbell or a weight plate with both hands. Squat down and twist to your right, attempting to touch the weight to the floor behind your right heel. Your left heel should come off the floor as you lower the weight to the floor. Then, as fast as you can, drive the weight back upward and across, finishing with the weight above and behind your left shoulder. Perform all of your reps on one side and then start on the other. The movement should resemble a corkscrew moving down into the ground and then moving back up.

Tip: *Bend at the knees as much as possible when lowering during the rotation so that the lower back doesn't absorb all of the stress of the movement.*

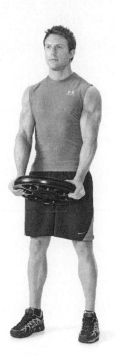

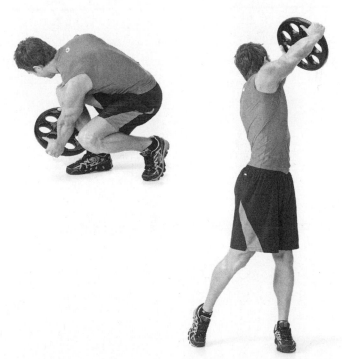

SWISS BALL WEIGHT ROLL

A good rotational movement that also requires the transverse abdominis to stabilize the torso.

Position yourself on a Swiss ball with your head and shoulders resting on the ball and feet walked out so that your torso is parallel with the floor. Holding a weight above your chest, rotate as far as possible to your right while attempting to maintain the position of your hips. Rotate until the outside of your shoulder is on the ball (you will feel as if you are about to roll off the ball). After decelerating the weight, forcefully drive back up and over to the other side.

Tip: Focus on contracting the glutes to keep the hips up at a constant level during the entire exercise, as they will tend to drop as the set proceeds.

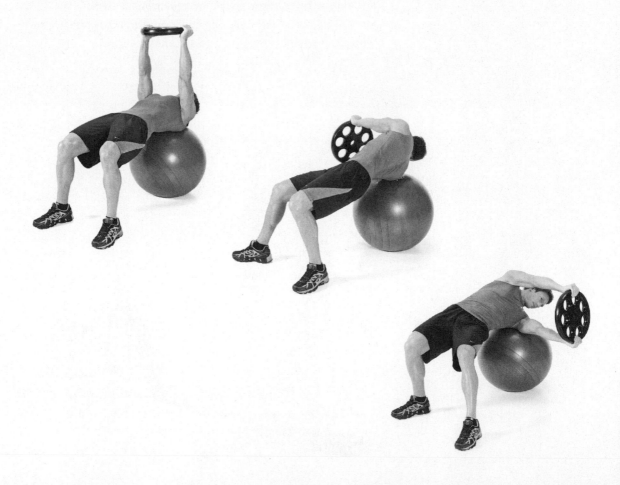

BARBELL TORQUE

Another rotational exercise that requires a large group of muscles to work in unison. This is a tremendous full-body exercise that will help develop an extremely strong core region.

Tip: *Keep in mind that the farther you extend your arms, the tougher the exercise will be.*

Place an Olympic bar in a wall corner. Place a towel in the corner to avoid damaging the walls or the bar. Place a weight (you may not need to add any weight when first attempting this exercise) on the end of the bar and hold it up at arm's length. Set your base a little wider than shoulder width and lean slightly forward into the weight. Rotate to your right as you start to lower the load down and outside your right knee. Your left heel will rise off the floor as you lower and your shoulders should follow your hands. Forcefully raise the weight back up and over to the other side and repeat.

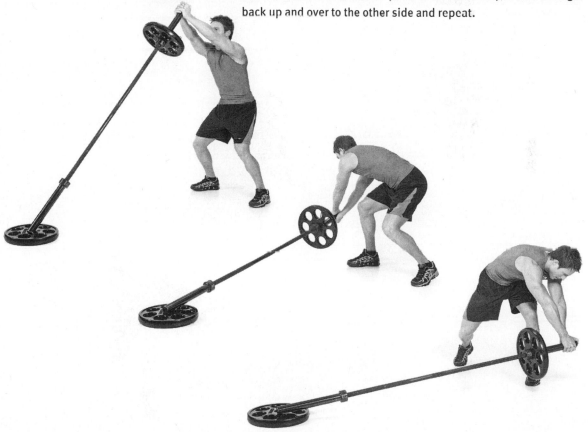

WINDSHIELD WIPER

This is one of the rotational exercises performed on the floor. It's a great exercise not only for developing rotational strength but also for promoting mobility as a result of the range of motion.

Lying on your back on the floor, lift your feet off the ground and hold your hips and knees at 90-degree angles. With your arms out to the sides for stabilization, rotate your thighs to the right until the outer thigh touches the ground. Keeping the knees together the entire time, rotate them back to the other side.

Tip: *There are three difficulty levels with this exercise. The easiest is feet up but close to the hips, the next is feet up with knees at 90 degrees (as in the exercise pictures), and the toughest is legs straight up so that the body resembles an "L."*

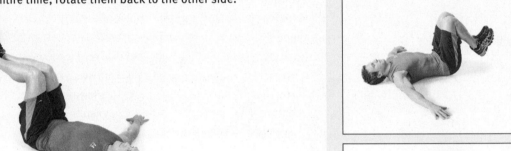

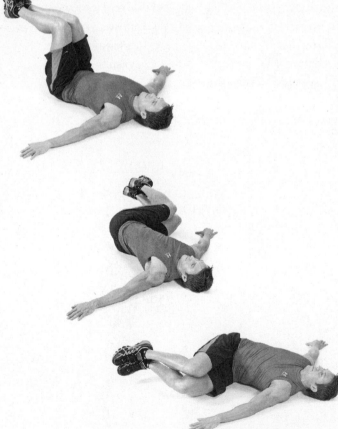

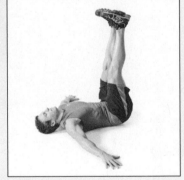

CABLE ROTATION

This ground-based rotational exercise is a highly effective core-strengthening movement. By recruiting strength that originates from the ground and moves through to the hands, this movement could easily be considered the king of rotational exercises.

Stand with feet slightly wider than shoulder width. Holding the cable handle out in front of your body at rib-cage level, rotate as far as possible to your left until you feel the muscles on your back right side begin to stretch. Drive back in the other direction, keeping your arms extended. Keep rotating until you feel the cable wrap around the back of your shoulder. Try to keep your feet stationary and drive the weight through the concentric phase (moving the load away from the weight stack) as fast as possible while returning the weight (eccentric) in a controlled manner. The exercise should resemble taking a home-run baseball swing.

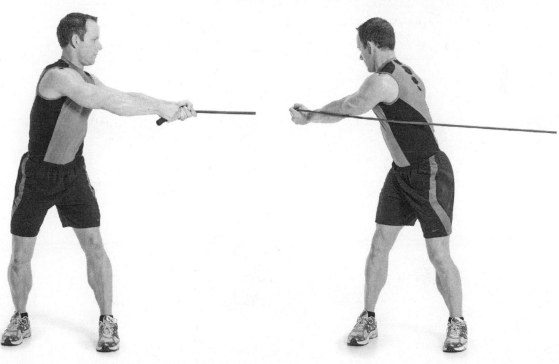

CABLE REVERSE WOOD CHOP

Similar to the cable rotation with the difference being an upward movement as you rotate. You will be a little weaker in this movement than the regular rotation due to raising the load. I prefer using a rope attachment with this exercise because it has a little more natural grip, and the two individual handles help emphasize that both hands are pulling equally.

Same setup as the cable rotation. As you lower the weight to the starting position, make sure to rotate as much as possible. As you bend your knees, lean forward at the hips. Drive back in the other direction, keeping your arms extended and aiming for a spot above your head (at arm's length). As with the cable rotation, rotate until you feel the cable across your shoulder.

Tip: *Keep your arms extended as much as possible so the cable doesn't come in contact with your face.*

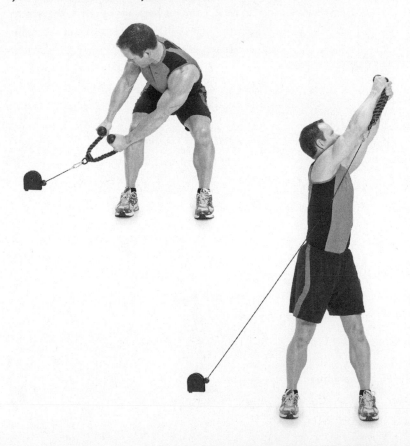

CABLE WOOD CHOP

Tip: *Keep your arms extended as much as possible so the cable doesn't come in contact with your face.*

The last of the cable rotation exercises, this targets rotation with a downward, chopping motion. You will be a little stronger on this exercise compared to the other cable exercises simply due to the addition of trunk flexion. As with the reverse cable wood chop, I recommend a rope attachment for this exercise.

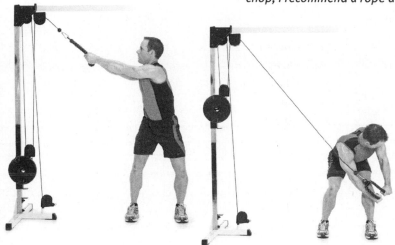

Use the same setup as the other cable rotations. As you raise the weight to the starting position, make sure to rotate as much as possible as you extend your legs and stretch upward. Rotate back in the other direction, keeping your arms extended and aiming for a spot below your knee (at arm's length). As with the other cable rotations, you should rotate until you feel the cable across the shoulder.

CABLE ROTATION VARIATIONS

Try these two cable rotation variations, as they tend to target the torso more than the standing variations. By taking the legs out of the movement, we can isolate the core region to a greater extent.

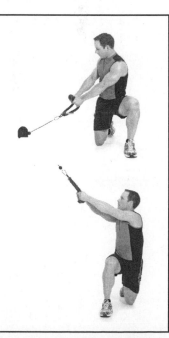

Kneeling Reverse Wood Chop

This exercise is almost identical to the standing version, only now you will be on one knee. Place the knee closest to the weight stack on the ground.

Kneeling Wood Chop

Again, this is almost identical to the standing version, only you will be on one knee. Place the knee farther away from the weight stack on the ground. Pull the load all the way to the floor each rep.

CABLE ROTATING CRUNCH

Using a rope attachment and the cable set at its highest level, face the cable stack. With arms extended and body upright, pull the rope handles down and to one side as you crunch down at the torso. Attempt to rotate as far as possible, facing the cable stack. Repeat on the other side.

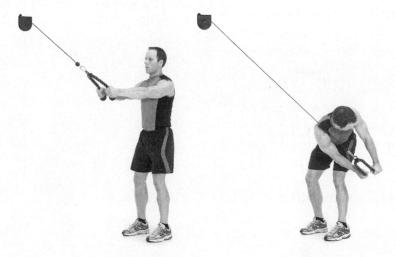

CABLE ROTATING EXTENSION

Use a rope attachment and the cable set at the lowest position. With arms in front of you, pull the rope up and to one side as you attempt to pull the weight up as high as possible and rotate as far as possible. Repeat on the other side.

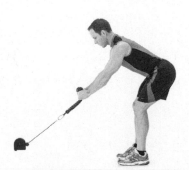
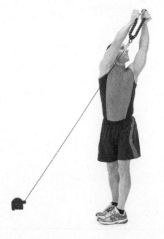

CABLE PUSH-PULL ROTATION

Tip: *Don't have access to cable resistance equipment? No problem. Try using one of these J.C. Bands that come in resistances ranging from easy to EXTREMELY difficult! These bands have two handles that require both arms to do equal amounts of work, and they can easily attach to a squat rack or other stable equipment. You can find these J.C. Bands at performbetter.com.*

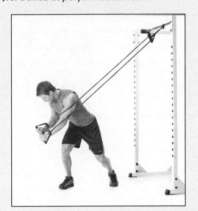

Stand between two cable stacks holding one handle in each hand with the cables set at waist height. Turn to your left so that your left arm is extended and your right hand is holding the handle at your chest. Your left foot should be staggered forward with your right leg back. Pull with your left hand as you push with your right hand, attempting to rotate the shoulders as far as possible. Repeat on the other side by simply turning the other direction, so that you will now be pulling/pushing with the opposite arms.

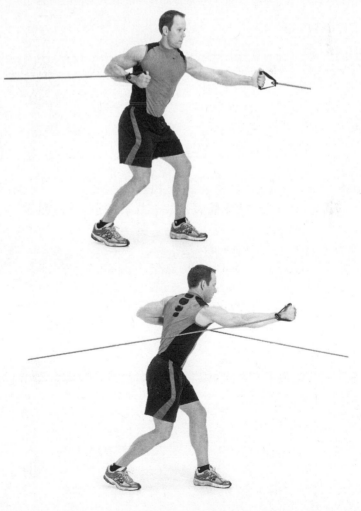

MEDICINE BALL STANDING WALL THROW

As mentioned earlier, the advantage to all of these medicine ball exercises is that you do not have to decelerate since you are letting go of the load. This enables us to generate a great deal of power during each throw. Try to regularly incorporate some of these effective medicine ball exercises, performing them against a wall or with a partner.

Standing with feet shoulder-width apart and shoulders perpendicular to a wall or a partner, rotate to your left as far as possible and swing back to your right to throw the ball as hard as you can either against a wall or to a partner. If using a wall, it helps to have a hard rubber medicine ball instead of a soft one, as it will bounce back with more velocity. As the ball comes back toward your hands, catch it and decelerate the load as you rotate back to your left to start another throw. If using a partner, have him throw the ball back to you as hard as possible, as this will add to the deceleration load.

> **Tip:** *Make sure not to pause during the deceleration phase; rather, using your body's stretch reflex, take advantage of the added power that you are able to generate. Also, try to gather all of your power from your legs and hips, as this will allow you to rotate even more.*

MEDICINE BALL OVER-THE-SHOULDER THROW AND CATCH

This unique exercise can also be done with a partner or with a wall. Its benefits are twofold: You'll get the uninhibited rotational throw, as well as a tremendous eccentric rotational load that you must decelerate to control the movement.

Standing with feet shoulder-width apart and back toward a wall or partner, rotate down and to your left until the ball is by your knee. Explosively rotate in the other direction as you rise, releasing the ball as you look over your shoulder. As the ball comes back to you (either rebounding off the wall or from a partner's throw), concentrate on slowing the ball down as you move back down into the starting position. Do not pause between the eccentric and concentric phases.

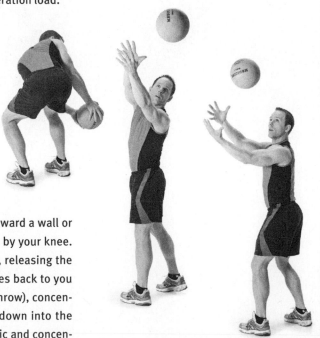

MEDICINE BALL 1-2-3 THROW

This exercise is a combination of a Russian twist with an uninhibited throw at the end of the movement—a great example of both a strength and power exercise.

Sitting perpendicular to a wall or a partner, lean back until your abs engage to stabilize your body. Perform three Russian twists as fast as possible by rotating outward first. You will be touching the ball to the ground in an outside-inside-outside sequence. After the final outside touch, release the ball by throwing it as hard as possible against the wall or to a partner—this is 1 repetition. As the ball comes back to you, immediately go back to the 1-2-3 Russian twist pattern.

Tip: As with Russian twists, make sure you lean back to engage your abs and force the rotational load during the entire exercise. To make the exercise more difficult, lean back and pick your feet up off the floor, keeping them off the floor for the duration of the exercise.

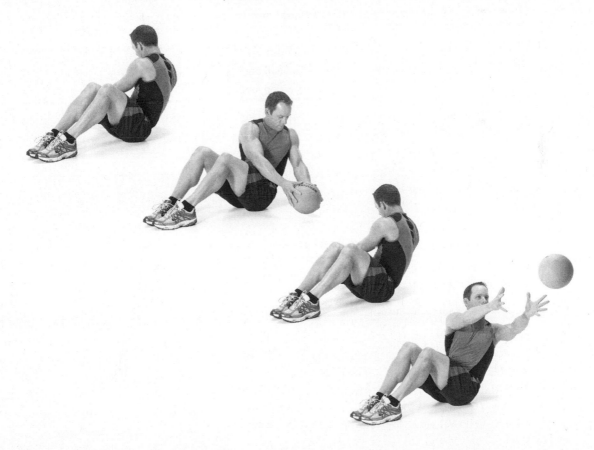

BRIDGING AND CORE STABILIZATION EXERCISES

Once again we will target the core with a variety of bridging-style exercises that force the transverse abdominis to forcefully contract in order to stabilize the body. This muscle group essentially wraps around the spine and supports the internal organs along with stabilizing the spine during static or dynamic movement. To get an idea of the area you're about to work, put your fingers around your waist and squeeze down. Now cough. You will feel the transverse abdominis (TVA) contract. Another way to feel them contract is to stand tall and try to squeeze your navel toward your spine as you exhale. The importance of this muscle group is quite significant when it comes to everyday activities like sitting tall, throwing a ball, running, performing squats, and so forth. The bottom line is that weak TVAs will result in weak performance when lifting or running around. When performing these bridging-style exercises, be sure to focus on keeping the TVA tight and stable throughout. While we often perform these bridging-style exercises in a static (motionless) fashion, I will also include dynamic options for many of them. By adding movement to the bridge, we can elicit greater core load and stimulate greater strength and stability development.

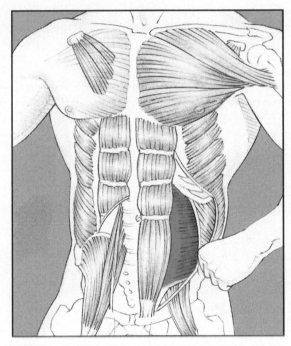

Bridging and core stabilization exercises target the transverse abdominis.

161

FOUR-POINT PLANK

Ah, yes! One of the most commonly seen exercises performed in gyms all over the world. This is a great exercise and one that will expose your TVA strength and endurance almost immediately.

Start on your stomach lying on the floor. Prop up onto your elbows, making sure to keep them lined up under your shoulders. Feet should be about shoulder-width apart with toes on the ground. Lift your hips off the floor and try to keep your shoulders, hips, and legs aligned (hips should not be too high or too low). Concentrate on pressing the navel into the spine while maintaining a relaxed breathing pattern. Keep the head in a neutral position during the exercise as you look at the floor. Most of these bridging exercises are determined by time rather than reps, so start with 15-second sets and gradually work your way up by adding 10 seconds each week or so.

Tip: *If you are unable to hold this plank position for 15 seconds, try performing this exercise on your elbows and knees rather than elbows and toes. Also, as you get stronger, try sliding your elbows farther forward to create less stability.*

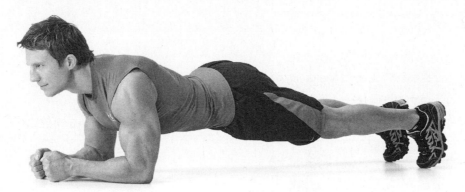

SHOULDERS HURT DURING PLANKS?

Some people experience some shoulder discomfort during planks. If this is the case, try performing the planks from an extended-arm position (like a pushup).

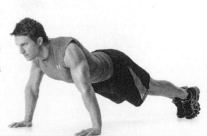

THREE-POINT PLANK

Same plank exercise with the difference being to create a less-stable environment by removing one of the contact points.

From the standard plank position, lift one foot off the ground approximately 6 inches. Try to hold the body in a perfect, stable position without tilting one way or the other. Alternate the raised leg every 10 seconds or so until you reach your total time goal.

The next progression in difficulty is to keep your feet on the floor and try to lift one arm. When doing this, try to maintain a level position at the shoulders, as there will be a tendency to lean one way or the other when your arm is off the ground. Trying to reach the arm out straight in front of you will limit tilting during the exercise. Alternate arms every 10 seconds or so.

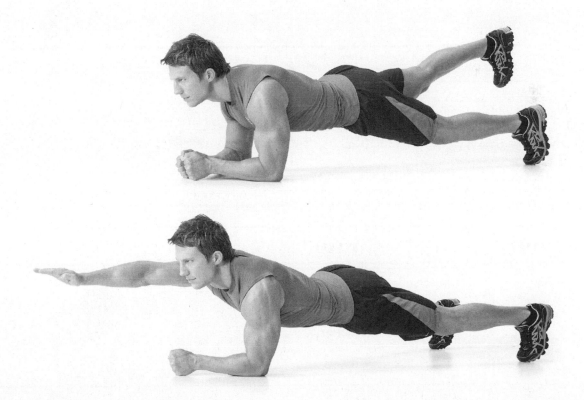

TWO-POINT PLANK

This is the same plank exercise as the four-point with the difference being that you will create an even greater instability by removing two points of contact.

From the standard plank position, lift one foot off the ground while picking up the opposite arm. Your hips may rise as you decrease the stability so try to keep your hips flat and look outward rather than downward during the exercise. Alternate arms and legs every 10 seconds or so.

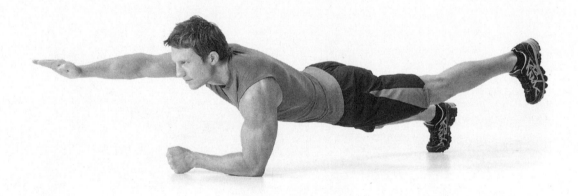

SIDE BRIDGE

This is a great core stabilization exercise that forces you to stabilize. As with the standard plank exercise, you can do this from the knees if you are unable to hold the elbow-foot position for more than 10 seconds or so.

Lying on your side, prop up on your elbow and forearm, making sure to keep your elbow lined up below your shoulder. Stack your feet on top of each other so that you are resting on the outside of the bottom foot. Pick your hips up and keep your upper hand on your hip. Look straight ahead so that your top shoulder doesn't roll forward. Try to keep as straight as possible during this exercise. There are several levels of difficulty and two different hand placements for this exercise.

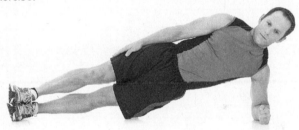

FEET

Level 1 is to rest on the elbow and the knees. Level 2 is to stagger your feet forward and back to add stability. Level 3 is to stack the feet on top of each other (as shown above). To further the challenge, you can start with the feet stacked and then lift the top foot off the bottom foot so you are holding it a few inches up in the air during the exercise.

ARM POSITION

The first position is on your elbow and forearm as described above. The second position is to place your hand on the ground and extend your arm so that you are holding this side bridge at arm's length. You can use all the earlier mentioned foot placement options from this extended position as well.

FOUR-POINT SUPINE BRIDGE

This is a commonly neglected bridging position. In this position we get tremendous transverse abdominis activation plus activation of the entire posterior chain. This exercise can be performed with two arm positions as well.

Starting faceup on the ground, prop up on your elbows as if you are picking up your shoulders to look at your feet. Keep your feet about shoulder-width apart with the back of your shoes on the ground and legs almost completely extended (bending your knees too much will result in a very easy exercise). Looking up to the ceiling, drive into the ground and lift your hips by contracting your hamstrings, glutes, and lower back. Hold this position.

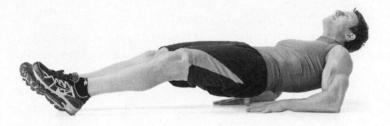

ARM POSITION

Arms can either be placed at your sides with weight on the elbows and forearms (as shown above) or at arm's length.

THREE-POINT SUPINE BRIDGE

This is the same bridge exercise as the previous exercise except that you will create a less-stable environment for yourself by lifting one of your feet.

From the supine bridge position, lift one foot off the ground approximately 6 inches. Attempt to hold your body in a perfect, stable position without tilting one way or the other. Alternate the raised leg every 10 seconds or so until you reach your total time goal.

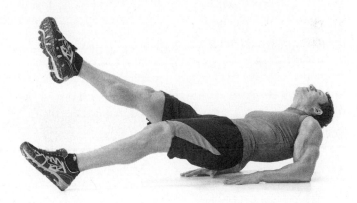

DYNAMIC PLANK

This is the same as the standard plank exercise but now we will add some movement to create greater stress on the core.

Holding a standard plank position, start to raise your hips as high as possible. At the highest point, lower your hips to the starting position. Continue this up-and-down movement for your goal time. Be sure you don't let your hips drop too low, as this will start to unnecessarily stress the lower back.

Tip: *Be sure to control this movement throughout the entire exercise, as there is a tendency to try to move faster to avoid the discomfort associated with slower movements.*

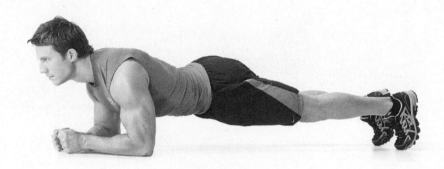

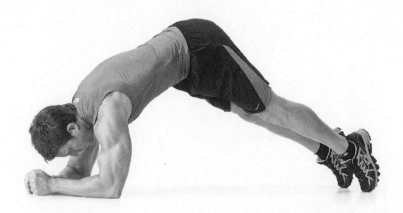

PLANK WITH ELBOW TO KNEE

In a standard plank position slowly, move your left elbow off the floor and down toward your right knee as you try to bring your right knee to meet halfway. Alternate elbows and knees.

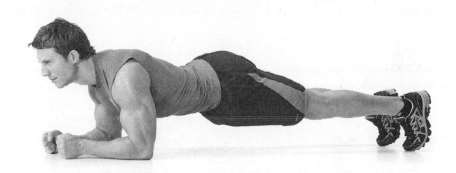

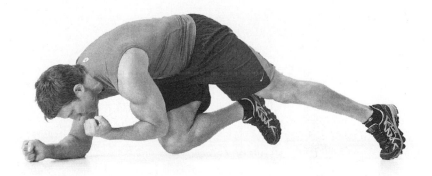

PLANK WALKUP

This is one of my favorite plank variations because it really focuses on stabilization during a very difficult movement pattern. The key to success for this exercise is to avoid a rolling motion of your torso during the walkups. Try to imagine you are balancing something on your lower back and any excessive movement will cause it to fall off. Remember to avoid leading with the same arm every single rep, as this will cause too much fatigue in one arm. Either alternate your lead arm or change arms every 10 seconds or so.

Start in the standard plank position. From here, walk your body up to a pushup position, pausing at the top for approximately 1 second. Lower your body back to the plank position and hold this position for 1 second as well. Continue to walk up and down for your goal time.

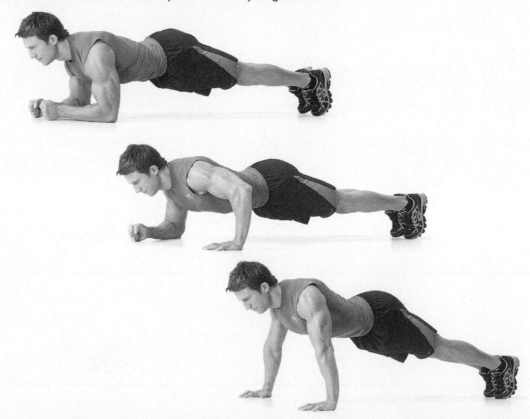

PLANK WITH WEIGHT TRANSFER

Tip: *Keep in mind that slower is tougher when it comes to this exercise!*

In a regular plank position, place a small weight plate on the ground outside your right elbow. Slowly pick up the weight with your right hand and pass it to your left hand. Then place the weight on the ground on your left side. Pause for a count before moving the weight back to the other side. Attempt to lift your elbow off the floor as you move the weight back and forth.

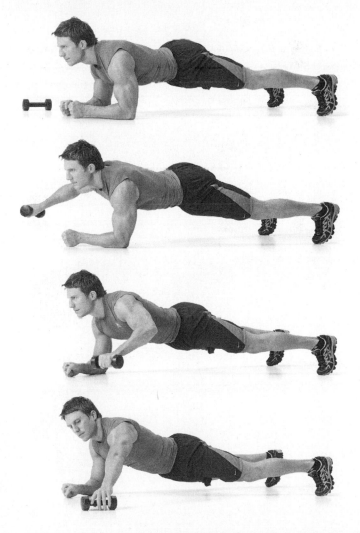

SIDE BRIDGE AND REACH

This exercise is an absolute killer! The key is to extend as far as possible during the reach phase while keeping only your arm and feet in contact with the floor.

Start in a side bridge position. Stretch your top arm up in the air and stabilize your body. Now reach down in front and then underneath your body as if you are trying to pick up a quarter off the floor behind you. Your shoulders should twist and now be parallel with the floor as you look back toward your fingers as they reach. Pause in this reach position for a second or two and return your arm to the out-stretched starting position. Perform these reaches for the goal amount of time, then switch to the other side.

Tip: These can be performed from any of the foot-placement positions mentioned earlier. Furthermore, adding a small weight to the reach hand will make the exercise even more difficult.

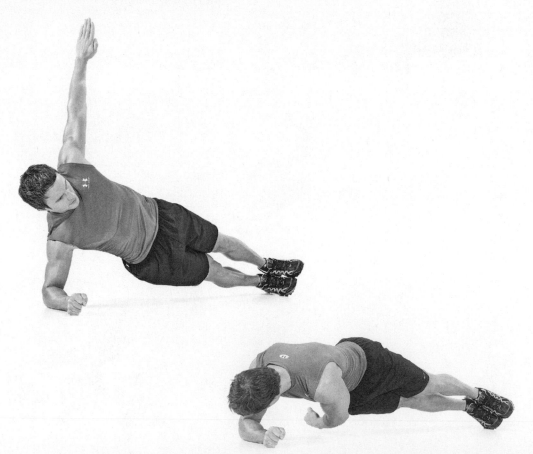

CORE ROW

This is yet another variation of a standard prone bridge. The addition of the rowing motion will force your core to stabilize to avoid tipping over. Try to keep your feet in contact with the ground during the row, as the opposite foot tends to rise off the ground when the opposite arm rows the weight.

Get into a pushup position while holding a pair of dumbbells with your feet shoulder-width apart. Keeping your body straight and without too much movement, row one dumbbell up until it touches your rib cage. Lower it back down, trying to set it as gently as possible on the floor. Repeat with the other dumbbell.

Tip: *If this exercise is too difficult, use lighter weights and/or set your feet wider apart. When performed correctly, this exercise should look as if the only thing moving during the rowing sequence is your arm.*

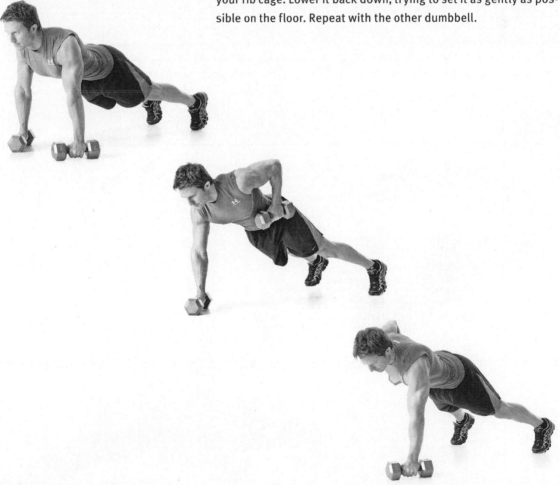

T-PUSH AND HOLD

This hybrid exercise combines a pushup with a side-bridge hold. There are three levels of difficulty for this exercise. Level 1 is with feet staggered during the side hold (as shown below). Level 2 is feet stacked during the hold, and level 3 is with the upper leg in the air during the hold. This is a difficult exercise that requires a tremendous amount of core stability for correct performance.

In a pushup position, lower into the pushup and drive back up to the side so that you finish on your right hand with the outside of your right foot on the ground and feet staggered. Your body should resemble the letter "T," as both arms will be extended and your torso will be rigid and stable. Pushing too hard out of the pushup will result in too much momentum into the bridge, while an insufficient push will not allow you to get all the way into the proper hold position.

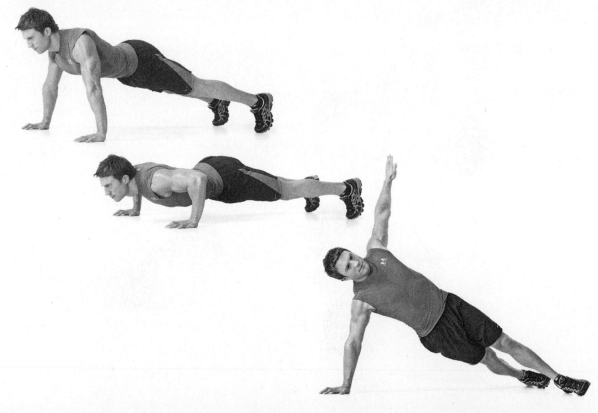

BARBELL ROLLOUT

This is a variation of the popular "ab roller"–style devices you see on TV. No fancy equipment is needed here, however, as you will use a standard barbell. This exercise will target the TVA along with the rectus abdominis due to the truck extension and flexion, which are essentially the movements we see during a situp. It is important to move slowly through this exercise to incorporate maximum core work.

With a barbell on the ground, set up on your knees and grab the bar with a shoulder-width pronated grip. Start with the bar close to your thighs. Push the bar forward, making sure to lead with the hands and follow with the hips (keeping the hips pushed back will result in less core stimulation). Roll out as far as possible, pausing for a second in the farthest position. Contract the abdominals and pull with the arms to start the movement back toward the starting position.

Tip: *Let your feet come up in the air as the bar moves forward. Also, try to experiment with the grip to find the most comfortable position for your shoulders.*

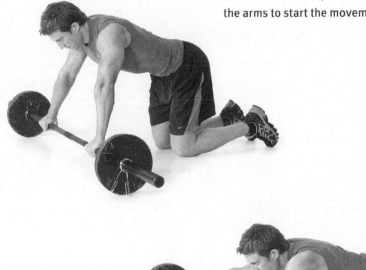

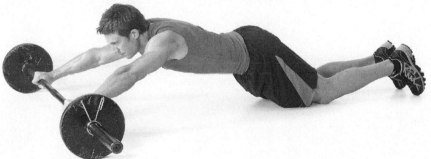

WARMUP COMPLEXES

The warmup complexes described in this chapter are a vital part of the *Men's Health* Power Training program. These exercises not only promote increased bloodflow and range of motion (as mentioned in Chapter 5), the specificity of movement patterns prepare your body for specific exercises. Most of the exercise patterns in the complexes are very similar to those used throughout the training programs.

Complexes are a series of exercises performed back-to-back, continuously without resting. You will complete all set reps of one exercise before moving onto the next exercise. These complexes are generally performed using an empty standard Olympic bar, which normally weighs 20 kilograms or sometimes 45 pounds (or lighter if needed) for 1 set of 5 to 8 repetitions. For the dumbbell complex sequence, I suggest using dumbbells no heavier than 25 pounds. Each of the three Power Training warmup complexes consists of six different movement patterns (exercises). As each of the exercises is described in the warmup complexes, a reference to where each can be found in the book accompanies. If an exercise is not in the menu categories, a short description is provided.

BARBELL COMPLEX

This complex consists of six exercises, all of which start from a hang position, as described in Chapter 8.

1. Hang Jump Shrug. Perform 5 jump shrugs, making sure to forcefully rise onto your toes and get complete "quadruple extension"—the simultaneous forceful extension of the ankles, knees, hips, and lower back—for each repetition. Detailed exercise description found on page 49.

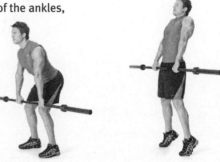

2. Hang Power Clean. Following the last hang jump shrug, perform 5 power cleans from the hang position, catching the weight and pausing at the top of each lift. Detailed exercise description found on page 55.

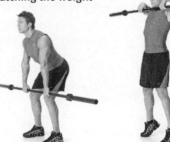
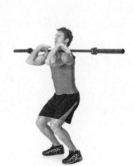

3. Push Press. Following the last hang power clean repetition, keep the bar at the shoulders and perform 5 explosive push presses. Detailed exercise description found on page 99.

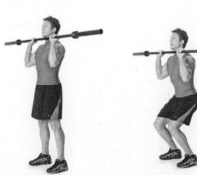

4. Front Squat. Following the last push press repetition, open your fingers so the bar is resting on the shoulders with elbows high. Perform 5 deep front squats. Detailed exercise description found on page 62.

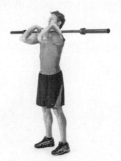 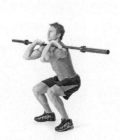

5. Bent-Over Row. Once the last front squat repetition is completed, bring the bar back down and position yourself for a wide-grip, bent-over row. Perform 5 of them. Detailed exercise description found on page 134.

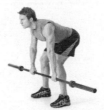 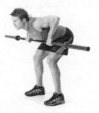

6. Romanian Deadlift. Finally, position your body for a slow set of 5 Romanian deadlifts, making sure to get a full range of motion. Detailed exercise description found on page 85.

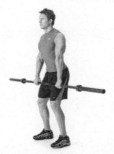 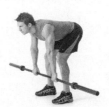

DUMBBELL COMPLEX

This warmup complex consists of six exercises, all performed with dumbbells and starting from a hang position.

1. Dumbbell High Pull. Perform 5 dumbbell high pulls, making sure to start each pull in a good "looking out the window" position you learned about on page 51. Once again, the quadruple extension is key in this movement.

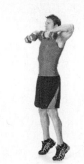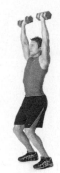

2. Hang Snatch. Following the last dumbbell high pull, perform 5 dumbbell snatches, emphasizing the extension and shrugging motion before driving the weights overhead. Detailed exercise description found on page 57.

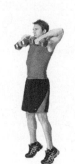

3. Squat and Press. Following the last dumbbell hang snatch, place the dumbbells on your shoulders, descend into a deep squat, and drive the weights overhead as you reach the top end of the squat. Perform 5 reps. Detailed exercise description found on page 236.

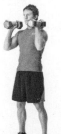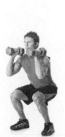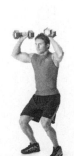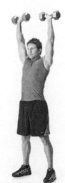

4. Bent-Over Alternating Row. Following the last dumbbell squat and press, bring the weights back down and perform 5 bent-over alternating rows with each arm. Detailed exercise description found on page 140.

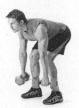 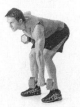 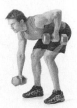

5. Pushup. Following the last set of dumbbell bent-over alternating rows, place the dumbbells on the ground and perform 5 pushups with your hands gripping the dumbbells on the ground. Detailed exercise description found on page 123.

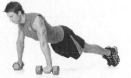 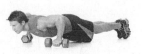

6. Core Row. Following the last pushup, stabilize the torso in a solid bridge and perform 5 core rows with each arm in alternating fashion. Detailed exercise description found on page 173.

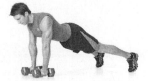 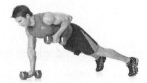

ADVANCED BARBELL COMPLEX

1. Hang Muscle Snatch. Perform 5 muscle snatches, emphasizing the shrug and the hips to move the bar into the press. Detailed exercise description found on page 57.

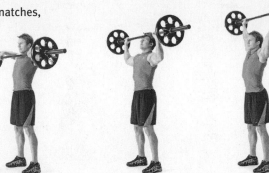
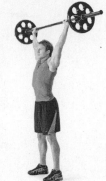

2. Overhead Squat. Setting the bar overhead, set your core and perform 5 deep overhead squats, pausing at the top of each repetition. Detailed exercise description found on page 64.

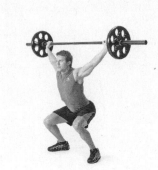

3. Snatch Drop Balance. Sit the bar on the back of your shoulders with hands in a wide-snatch grip. With your feet in a jumping base as described on page 45, dip at the knees and drive under the weight, trying to keep the bar at the same height as where it started on your shoulders. As you drive under the bar, your feet will spread out to a catching base as your elbows lock out the bar overhead. Stand to an upright position before lowering the bar to your shoulders for the next repetition. Perform 5 reps.

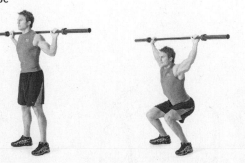

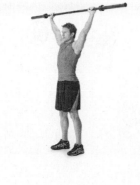
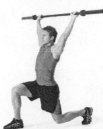

4. Overhead Lunge. Press the weight overhead using a snatch grip. Perform 5 forward lunges on each leg, keeping the torso erect and eyes up.

5. Squat Hang Clean. This is very similar to a standard hang clean with the exception that it is more like a hybrid because of the front squat. As you catch the weight at the shoulders, immediately descend into a deep front squat. There is no pause after catching the weight. Think of it as if you catch the load and the load forces your body down into the squat. Perform 5 reps.

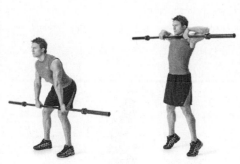
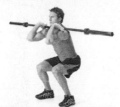

6. Bent-Over Row and Back Extension. This is the hybrid lift described in detail on page 248. From the bent-over position, perform the row, pin the weight to your chest, and perform the back extension. Reverse the movements, making sure to keep the weight pinned to your chest until it is time to extend your arms back down to begin the next rep. Perform 5 reps.

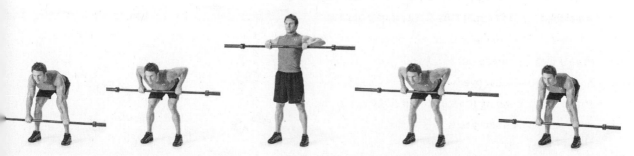

PART 4

THE POWER TRAINING WORKOUTS

TOTAL FITNESS TRAINING

The purpose of the total fitness training program is to develop a well-rounded program that alternates between higher-volume (more sets/reps), moderate-load cycles and lower-volume, higher-intensity training cycles. The results will be a total package of increased muscle size and increased muscular strength. The sample programs found in this chapter highlight both full-body and push-pull routines.

Keep in mind that the majority of trainees will feel most comfortable with this routine as it allows for a significant change in volumes and loads every 3 weeks. This program is also best suited for those who want to improve total fitness rather than those who want to focus on muscle size or muscle strength gains.

Average repetitions performed per exercise

Weeks 1 to 3 = 40

Weeks 4 to 6 = 24

Weeks 7 to 9 = 32

Weeks 10 to 12 = 16

Rest periods

Explosive Exercises = 90 seconds to 2 minutes

1 to 6 reps = 90 seconds to 2 minutes

8 to 12 reps = 60 seconds

Complexing allowed = YES

Unloading recommendations = At least one to two sessions every 6 weeks

SAMPLE 3-DAY FULL-BODY WORKOUT FOR TOTAL FITNESS TRAINING (WEEKS 1–3)

WEEK 1

MOVEMENT	EXERCISE	1	2	3	4
	WORKOUT A				
EXPLOSIVE	HANG POWER CLEAN	/5	/5	/5	/5
KNEE DOMINANT	FRONT SQUAT	/10	/10	/10	/10
HIP DOMINANT	1-LEG ROM DEADLIFT	/10	/10	/10	/10
HORIZONTAL PUSH	BENCH PRESS	/10	/10	/10	/10
HORIZONTAL PULL	DB ROW	/10	/10	/10	/10
VERTICAL PUSH	PUSH PRESS	/10	/10	/10	/10
VERTICAL PULL	1-ARM LAT PLDWN	/10	/10	/10	/10
ROTATIONAL	SEATED RUSS TWIST	/10	/10	/10	/10
BRIDGING	PLANK ELBOW TO KNEE	30–45 sec	30–45 sec	30–45 sec	30–45 sec

WEEK 2

MOVEMENT	EXERCISE	1	2	3	4
	WORKOUT B				
EXPLOSIVE	MUSCLE SNATCH	/5	/5	/5	/5
KNEE DOMINANT	1-LEG SQUAT	/10	/10	/10	/10
HIP DOMINANT	ROM DEADLIFT	/10	/10	/10	/10
HORIZONTAL PUSH	DB 1-ARM ON BALL	/10	/10	/10	/10
HORIZONTAL PULL	CABLE FACE PULL	/10	/10	/10	/10
VERTICAL PUSH	DB SPLIT JERK	/10	/10	/10	/10
VERTICAL PULL	CHINUP	/10	/10	/10	/10
ROTATIONAL	PARALLEL SWING	/10	/10	/10	/10
BRIDGING	DYNAMIC PLANK	30–45 sec	30–45 sec	30–45 sec	30–45 sec

WEEK 3

MOVEMENT	EXERCISE	1	2	3	4
	WORKOUT A				
EXPLOSIVE	DB SNATCH	/5	/5	/5	/5
KNEE DOMINANT	OVRHD SQUAT	/10	/10	/10	/10
HIP DOMINANT	1-LEG BACK EXT	/10	/10	/10	/10
HORIZONTAL PUSH	INCLINE BENCH PRESS	/10	/10	/10	/10
HORIZONTAL PULL	DB ROW	/10	/10	/10	/10
VERTICAL PUSH	PUSH JERK	/10	/10	/10	/10
VERTICAL PULL	SIDE-TO-SIDE PULLUP	/10	/10	/10	/10
ROTATIONAL	REV WOOD CHOP	/10	/10	/10	/10
BRIDGING	SUPINE BRIDGE	30–45 sec	30–45 sec	30–45 sec	30–45 sec

EXERCISE	1	2	3	4	EXERCISE	1	2	3	4
WORKOUT B					**WORKOUT A**				
HANG JUMP SHRUG	/5	/5	/5	/5	SNATCH PULL	/5	/5	/5	/5
DROP LUNGE	/10	/10	/10	/10	SPLIT SQUAT	/10	/10	/10	
GOOD MORN	/10	/10	/10	/10	1-LEG BACK EXT	/10	/10	/10	
DB INCLINE BENCH PRESS	/10	/10	/10	/10	REV-GRIP BENCH PRESS	/10	/10	/10	
HORIZ PULLUP	/10	/10	/10	/10	1-ARM CABLE ROW	/10	/10	/10	
SUPPORTED DB 1-ARM PRESS	/10	/10	/10	/10	PUSH JERK	/10	/10	/10	
WIDE-GRIP PULLUP	/10	/10	/10	/10	SIDE-TO-SIDE PULLUP	/10	/10	/10	
CORKSCREW	/10	/10	/10	/10	WOOD CHOP	/10	/10	/10	
PLANK	30–45 sec	30–45 sec	30–45 sec	30–45 sec	PLANK WALKUP	30–45 sec	30–45 sec	30–45 sec	30–45 sec

EXERCISE	1	2	3	4	EXERCISE	1	2	3	4
WORKOUT A					**WORKOUT B**				
HANG POWER SNATCH	/5	/5	/5	/5	DB HANG POWER CLEAN	/5	/5	/5	/5
BACK SQUAT	/10	/10	/10	/10	BULG SPLIT SQUAT	/10	/10	/10	
1-LEG GOOD MORN	/10	/10	/10	/10	ROM DEADLIFT	/10	/10	/10	
BENCH PRESS	/10	/10	/10	/10	DB INCLINE ON BALL	/10	/10	/10	
DB ROW + TWIST	/10	/10	/10	/10	CABLE ROW TO NECK	/10	/10	/10	
PUSH PRESS	/10	/10	/10	/10	DB PUSH JERK	/10	/10	/10	
1-ARM PLDWN	/10	/10	/10	/10	CHINUP	/10	/10	/10	
SWISS BALL WT ROLL	/10	/10	/10	/10	BB TORQUE	/10	/10	/10	
SIDE PLANK	30–45 sec	30–45 sec	30–45 sec	30–45 sec	PLANK W/ WT TRANS	30–45 sec	30–45 sec	30–45 sec	30–45 sec

EXERCISE	1	2	3	4	EXERCISE	1	2	3	4
WORKOUT B					**WORKOUT A**				
CLEAN PULL	/5	/5	/5	/5	POWER CLEAN	/5	/5	/5	/5
STEPUP	/10	/10	/10	/10	SPLIT SQUAT	/10	/10	/10	
SEATED GOOD MORN	/10	/10	/10	/10	1-LEG ROM DEADLIFT	/10	/10	/10	
SIDE-TO-SIDE PUSHUP	/10	/10	/10	/10	DIP	/10	/10	/10	
CABLE ROW	/10	/10	/10	/10	1-ARM CABLE ROW TO NECK	/10	/10	/10	
DB PUSH PRESS	/10	/10	/10	/10	SPLIT JERK	/10	/10	/10	
MIXED-GRIP PULLUP	/10	/10	/10	/10	SIDE-TO-SIDE PULLUP	/10	/10	/10	
WOOD CHOP KNEE	/10	/10	/10	/10	SEATED RUSS TWIST	/10	/10	/10	
SIDE PLANK REACH	30–45 sec	30–45 sec	30–45 sec	30–45 sec	PLANK WALKUP	30–45 sec	30–45 sec	30–45 sec	30–45 sec

SAMPLE 4-DAY PUSH-PULL WORKOUT FOR TOTAL FITNESS TRAINING (WEEKS 1–3)

WEEK 1

MOVEMENT	EXERCISE	1	2	3	4	EXERCISE	1	2	3	4	
	WORKOUT A1					WORKOUT B1					
EXPLOSIVE	CLEAN PULL	/5	/5	/5	/5	MUSCLE SNATCH	/5	/5	/5	/5	
HIP/KNEE DOMINANT	FRONT SQUAT	/10	/10	/10	/10	1-LEG ROM DEADLIFT	/10	/10	/10	/10	
HORIZONTAL PUSH/PULL	DB BENCH PRESS	/10	/10	/10	/10	CABLE FACE PULL	/10	/10	/10	/10	
VERTICAL PUSH/PULL	PUSH PRESS	/10	/10	/10	/10	1-ARM PLDWN	/10	/10	/10	/10	
ROTATIONAL	WOOD CHOP	/10	/10	/10	/10	SEATED RUSS TWIST	/10	/10	/10	/10	
BRIDGING	PLANK	30–45 sec	30–45 sec	30–45 sec	30–45 sec	SIDE PLANK + REACH	30–45 sec	30–45 sec	30–45 sec	30–45 sec	

WEEK 2

MOVEMENT	EXERCISE	1	2	3	4	EXERCISE	1	2	3	4	
	WORKOUT A1					WORKOUT B1					
EXPLOSIVE	DB SNATCH	/5	/5	/5	/5	HANG POWER CLEAN	/5	/5	/5	/5	
HIP/KNEE DOMINANT	SPLIT SQUAT	/10	/10	/10	/10	1-LEG BACK EXT	/10	/10	/10	/10	
HORIZONTAL PUSH/PULL	SIDE-TO-SIDE PUSHUP	/10	/10	/10	/10	HORIZ PULLUP	/10	/10	/10	/10	
VERTICAL PUSH/PULL	JACKKNIFE PUSHUP	/10	/10	/10	/10	SIDE-TO-SIDE PULLUP	/10	/10	/10	/10	
ROTATIONAL	CABLE PUSH-PULL ROT	/10	/10	/10	/10	MED BALL 1-2-3	/10	/10	/10	/10	
BRIDGING	SIDE PLANK	30–45 sec	30–45 sec	30–45 sec	30–45 sec	DYNAMIC PLANK	30–45 sec	30–45 sec	30–45 sec	30–45 sec	

WEEK 3

MOVEMENT	EXERCISE	1	2	3	4	EXERCISE	1	2	3	4	
	WORKOUT A1					WORKOUT B1					
EXPLOSIVE	CLEAN PULL	/5	/5	/5	/5	SNATCH PULL	/5	/5	/5	/5	
HIP/KNEE DOMINANT	BACK SQUAT	/10	/10	/10	/10	1-LEG GOOD MORN	/10	/10	/10	/10	
HORIZONTAL PUSH/PULL	DB INCLINE BENCH PRESS	/10	/10	/10	/10	BENT-OVR ROW	/10	/10	/10	/10	
VERTICAL PUSH/PULL	SPLIT JERK	/10	/10	/10	/10	1-ARM PLDWN	/10	/10	/10	/10	
ROTATIONAL	SWISS BALL WT ROLL	/10	/10	/10	/10	BB TORQUE	/10	/10	/10	/10	
BRIDGING	PLANK W/ ELBOW TO KNEE	30–45 sec	30–45 sec	30–45 sec	30–45 sec	PLANK W/ WT TRANS	30–45 sec	30–45 sec	30–45 sec	30–45 sec	

EXERCISE	1	2	3	4	EXERCISE	1	2	3	4
WORKOUT A2					WORKOUT B2				
DB HANG POWER CLEAN	/5	/5	/5	/5	NARROW-GRIP HANG SNATCH	/5	/5	/5	/5
STEPUP	/10	/10	/10	/10	ROM DEADLIFT	/10	/10	/10	/10
CLOSE-GRIP BENCH PRESS	/10	/10	/10	/10	DB ROW + TWIST	/10	/10	/10	/10
SUPPORTED DB 1-ARM PRESS	/10	/10	/10	/10	CHINUP	/10	/10	/10	/10
WINDSHIELD WIPER	/10	/10	/10	/10	REV WOOD CHOP KNEE	/10	/10	/10	/10
PLANK WALKUP	30–45 sec	30–45 sec	30–45 sec	30–45 sec	2-PT PLANK	30–45 sec	30–45 sec	30–45 sec	30–45 sec

EXERCISE	1	2	3	4	EXERCISE	1	2	3	4
WORKOUT A2					WORKOUT B2				
HANG JUMP SHRUG	/5	/5	/5	/5	CLEAN PULL	/5	/5	/5	/5
BULG SPLIT SQUAT	/10	/10	/10	/10	GOOD MORN	/10	/10	/10	/10
REV-GRIP BENCH PRESS	/10	/10	/10	/10	1-ARM CABLE ROW	/10	/10	/10	/10
DB PUSH PRESS	/10	/10	/10	/10	WIDE-GRIP PULLUP	/10	/10	/10	/10
CORKSCREW	/10	/10	/10	/10	CABLE PARALLEL	/10	/10	/10	/10
PLANK	30–45 sec	30–45 sec	30–45 sec	30–45 sec	SIDE PLANK+REACH	30–45 sec	30–45 sec	30–45 sec	30–45 sec

EXERCISE	1	2	3	4	EXERCISE	1	2	3	4
WORKOUT A2					WORKOUT B2				
HIGH PULL	/5	/5	/5	/5	HANG POWER CLEAN	/5	/5	/5	/5
1-LEG SQUAT	/10	/10	/10	/10	SEATED GOOD MORN	/10	/10	/10	/10
PUSHUP	/10	/10	/10	/10	HORIZ SIDE-TO-SIDE PULLUP	/10	/10	/10	/10
CABLE PRESS	/10	/10	/10	/10	LAT PLDWN	/10	/10	/10	/10
WOOD CHOP KNEE	/10	/10	/10	/10	MED BALL OVER SHOULDER	/10	/10	/10	/10
POST BRIDGE	30–45 sec	30–45 sec	30–45 sec	30–45 sec	CORE ROW	30–45 sec	30–45 sec	30–45 sec	30–45 sec

HYPERTROPHY TRAINING

The purpose of this hypertrophy training program is to develop as much muscle size as possible. Unlike the total fitness program, this program is characterized by much greater work volumes for its duration. While there will still be an alternating pattern every 3 weeks, the changes in volumes and loads will not be as significant as the total fitness program. The results for this particular training program will be greater muscle size gains but not necessarily greater 1-repetition maximum strength gains. The sample programs found in this chapter highlight both full-body and push-pull routines.

While it is okay to follow this program for the entire 12 weeks, I suggest you move back to the more traditional alternating periodization scheme (i.e., the total fitness program) after you complete the 12-week program. After a 12-week cycle with the total fitness program, you can come back to the hypertrophy program for another 12 weeks.

Average repetitions performed per exercise

Weeks 1 to 3 = 40

Weeks 4 to 6 = 32

Weeks 7 to 9 = 32

Weeks 10 to 12 = 36

Rest periods

Explosive Exercises = 90 seconds to 2 minutes

1 to 6 reps = 90 seconds to 2 minutes

8 to 12 reps = 60 seconds

Complexing allowed = YES

Unloading recommendations = At least one to two sessions every 6 weeks

SAMPLE 3-DAY FULL-BODY WORKOUT FOR HYPERTROPHY TRAINING (WEEKS 4–6)

WEEK 4

MOVEMENT	EXERCISE	1	2	3	4	
	WORKOUT A					
EXPLOSIVE	HANG POWER CLEAN	/3	/3	/3	/3	
KNEE DOMINANT	FRONT SQUAT	/10	/8	/8	/6	
HIP DOMINANT	1-LEG ROM DEADLIFT	/10	/8	/8	/6	
HORIZONTAL PUSH	BENCH PRESS	/10	/8	/8	/6	
HORIZONTAL PULL	DB ROW	/10	/8	/8	/6	
VERTICAL PUSH	PUSH PRESS	/10	/8	/8	/6	
VERTICAL PULL	1-ARM PLDWN	/10	/8	/8	/6	
ROTATIONAL	SEATED RUSS TWIST	/10	/10	/10	/10	
BRIDGING	PLANK ELBOW TO KNEE	30–45 sec	30–45 sec	30–45 sec	30–45 sec	

WEEK 5

MOVEMENT	EXERCISE	1	2	3	4	
	WORKOUT B					
EXPLOSIVE	MUSCLE SNATCH	/3	/3	/3	/3	
KNEE DOMINANT	1-LEG SQUAT	/10	/8	/8	/6	
HIP DOMINANT	ROM DEADLIFT	/10	/8	/8	/6	
HORIZONTAL PUSH	DB 1-ARM ON BALL	/10	/8	/8	/6	
HORIZONTAL PULL	CABLE FACE PULL	/10	/8	/8	/6	
VERTICAL PUSH	DB SPLIT JERK	/10	/8	/8	/6	
VERTICAL PULL	CHINUP	/10	/8	/8	/6	
ROTATIONAL	PARALLEL SWING	/10	/10	/10	/10	
BRIDGING	DYNAMIC PLANK	30–45 sec	30–45 sec	30–45 sec	30–45 sec	

WEEK 6

MOVEMENT	EXERCISE	1	2	3	4	
	WORKOUT A					
EXPLOSIVE	DB SNATCH	/3	/3	/3	/3	
KNEE DOMINANT	OVRHD SQUAT	/10	/8	/8	/6	
HIP DOMINANT	1-LEG BACK EXT	/10	/8	/8	/6	
HORIZONTAL PUSH	INCLINE BENCH	/10	/8	/8	/6	
HORIZONTAL PULL	DB ROW	/10	/8	/8	/6	
VERTICAL PUSH	PUSH JERK	/10	/8	/8	/6	
VERTICAL PULL	SIDE-TO-SIDE PULLUP	/10	/8	/8	/6	
ROTATIONAL	REV WOOD CHOP	/10	/10	/10	/10	
BRIDGING	SUPINE BRIDGE	30–45 sec	30–45 sec	30–45 sec	30–45 sec	

EXERCISE	1	2	3	4
WORKOUT B				
HANG JUMP SHRUG	/3	/3	/3	/3
DROP LUNGE	/10	/8	/8	/6
GOOD MORN	/10	/8	/8	/6
DB INCLINE BENCH PRESS	/10	/8	/8	/6
HORIZ PULLUP	/10	/8	/8	/6
SUPPORTED DB 1-ARM PRESS	/10	/8	/8	/6
WIDE-GRIP PULLUP	/10	/8	/8	/6
CORKSCREW	/10	/10	/10	/10
PLANK	30–45 sec	30–45 sec	30–45 sec	30–45 sec

EXERCISE	1	2	3	4
WORKOUT A				
SNATCH PULL	/3	/3	/3	/3
SPLIT SQUAT	/10	/8	/8	/6
1-LEG BACK EXT	/10	/8	/8	/6
REV-GRIP BENCH PRESS	/10	/8	/8	/6
1-ARM CABLE ROW	/10	/8	/8	/6
PUSH JERK	/10	/8	/8	/6
SIDE-TO-SIDE PULLUP	/10	/8	/8	/6
WOOD CHOP	/10	/10	/10	/10
PLANK WALKUP	30–45 sec	30–45 sec	30–45 sec	30–45 sec

EXERCISE	1	2	3	4
WORKOUT A				
HANG POWER SNATCH	/3	/3	/3	/3
BACK SQUAT	/10	/8	/8	/6
1-LEG GOOD MORN	/10	/8	/8	/6
BENCH PRESS	/10	/8	/8	/6
DB ROW + TWIST	/10	/8	/8	/6
PUSH PRESS	/10	/8	/8	/6
1-ARM PLDWN	/10	/8	/8	/6
SWISS BALL WT ROLL	/10	/10	/10	/10
SIDE PLANK	30–45 sec	30–45 sec	30–45 sec	30–45 sec

EXERCISE	1	2	3	4
WORKOUT B				
DB HANG POWER CLEAN	/3	/3	/3	/3
BULG SPLIT SQUAT	/10	/8	/8	/6
ROM DEADLIFT	/10	/8	/8	/6
DB INCLINE ON BALL	/10	/8	/8	/6
CABLE ROW TO NECK	/10	/8	/8	/6
DB PUSH JERK	/10	/8	/8	/6
CHINUP	/10	/8	/8	/6
BB TORQUE	/10	/10	/10	/10
PLANK W/ WT TRANS	30–45 sec	30–45 sec	30–45 sec	30–45 sec

EXERCISE	1	2	3	4
WORKOUT B				
CLEAN PULL	/3	/3	/3	/3
STEPUP	/10	/8	/8	/6
SEATED GOOD MORN	/10	/8	/8	/6
SIDE-TO-SIDE PUSHUP	/10	/8	/8	/6
CABLE ROW	/10	/8	/8	/6
DB PUSH PRESS	/10	/8	/8	/6
MIXED-GRIP PULLUP	/10	/8	/8	/6
WOOD CHOP KNEE	/10	/10	/10	/10
SIDE PLANK REACH	30–45 sec	30–45 sec	30–45 sec	30–45 sec

EXERCISE	1	2	3	4
WORKOUT A				
POWER CLEAN	/3	/3	/3	/3
SPLIT SQUAT	/10	/8	/8	/6
1-LEG ROM DEADLIFT	/10	/8	/8	/6
DIP	/10	/8	/8	/6
1-ARM CABLE ROW TO NECK	/10	/8	/8	/6
SPLIT JERK	/10	/8	/8	/6
SIDE-TO-SIDE PULLUP	/10	/8	/8	/6
SEATED RUSS TWIST	/10	/10	/10	/10
PLANK WALKUP	30–45 sec	30–45 sec	30–45 sec	30–45 sec

SAMPLE 4-DAY PUSH-PULL WORKOUT FOR HYPERTROPHY TRAINING (WEEKS 4–6)

WEEK 4

MOVEMENT	EXERCISE	1	2	3	4	EXERCISE	1	2	3	4
	WORKOUT A1					WORKOUT B1				
EXPLOSIVE	CLEAN PULL	/3	/3	/3	/3	MUSCLE SNATCH	/3	/3	/3	/3
HIP/KNEE DOMINANT	FRONT SQUAT	/10	/8	/8	/6	1-LEG ROM DEADLIFT	/10	/8	/8	/6
HORIZONTAL PUSH/PULL	DB BENCH PRESS	/10	/8	/8	/6	CABLE FACE PULL	/10	/8	/8	/6
VERTICAL PUSH/PULL	PUSH PRESS	/10	/8	/8	/6	1-ARM PLDWN	/10	/8	/8	/6
ROTATIONAL	WOOD CHOP	/10	/10	/10	/10	SEATED RUSS TWIST	/10	/10	/10	/10
BRIDGING	PLANK	30–45 sec	30–45 sec	30–45 sec	30–45 sec	SIDE PLANK + REACH	30–45 sec	30–45 sec	30–45 sec	30–45 sec

WEEK 5

MOVEMENT	EXERCISE	1	2	3	4	EXERCISE	1	2	3	4
	WORKOUT A1					WORKOUT B1				
EXPLOSIVE	DB SNATCH	/3	/3	/3	/3	HANG POWER CLEAN	/3	/3	/3	/3
HIP/KNEE DOMINANT	SPLIT SQUAT	/10	/8	/8	/6	1-LEG BACK EXT	/10	/8	/8	/6
HORIZONTAL PUSH/PULL	SIDE-TO-SIDE PUSHUP	/10	/8	/8	/6	HORIZ PULLUP	/10	/8	/8	/6
VERTICAL PUSH/PULL	JACKKNIFE PUSHUP	/10	/8	/8	/6	SIDE-TO-SIDE PULLUP	/10	/8	/8	/6
ROTATIONAL	CABLE PUSH-PULL ROT	/10	/10	/10	/10	MED BALL 1-2-3	/10	/10	/10	/10
BRIDGING	SIDE PLANK	30–45 sec	30–45 sec	30–45 sec	30–45 sec	DYNAMIC PLANK	30–45 sec	30–45 sec	30–45 sec	30–45 sec

WEEK 6

MOVEMENT	EXERCISE	1	2	3	4	EXERCISE	1	2	3	4
	WORKOUT A1					WORKOUT B1				
EXPLOSIVE	CLEAN PULL	/3	/3	/3	/3	SNATCH PULL	/3	/3	/3	/3
HIP/KNEE DOMINANT	BACK SQUAT	/10	/8	/8	/6	1-LEG GOOD MORN	/10	/8	/8	/6
HORIZONTAL PUSH/PULL	DB INCLINE BENCH PRESS	/10	/8	/8	/6	BENT-OVR ROW	/10	/8	/8	/6
VERTICAL PUSH/PULL	SPLIT JERK	/10	/8	/8	/6	1-ARM PLDWN	/10	/8	/8	/6
ROTATIONAL	SWISS BALL WT ROLL	/10	/10	/10	/10	BB TORQUE	/10	/10	/10	/10
BRIDGING	PLANK W/ ELBOW TO KNEE	30–45 sec	30–45 sec	30–45 sec	30–45 sec	PLANK W/ WT TRANS	30–45 sec	30–45 sec	30–45 sec	30–45 sec

EXERCISE	1	2	3	4	EXERCISE	1	2	3	4
WORKOUT A2					WORKOUT B2				
DB HANG POWER CLEAN	/3	/3	/3	/3	NARROW-GRIP HANG SNATCH	/3	/3	/3	/3
STEPUP	/10	/8	/8	/6	ROM DEADLIFT	/10	/8	/8	/6
CLOSE-GRIP BENCH PRESS	/10	/8	/8	/6	DB ROW + TWIST	/10	/8	/8	/6
SUPPORTED DB 1-ARM PRESS	/10	/8	/8	/6	CHINUP	/10	/8	/8	/6
WINDSHIELD WIPER	/10	/10	/10	/10	REV WOOD CHOP KNEE	/10	/10	/10	/10
PLANK WALKUP	30–45 sec	30–45 sec	30–45 sec	30–45 sec	2-PT PLANK	30–45 sec	30–45 sec	30–45 sec	30–45 sec

EXERCISE	1	2	3	4	EXERCISE	1	2	3	4
WORKOUT A2					WORKOUT B2				
HANG JUMP SHRUG	/3	/3	/3	/3	CLEAN PULL	/3	/3	/3	/3
BULG SPLIT SQUAT	/10	/8	/8	/6	GOOD MORN	/10	/8	/8	/6
REV-GRIP BENCH PRESS	/10	/8	/8	/6	1-ARM CABLE ROW	/10	/8	/8	/6
DB PUSH PRESS	/10	/8	/8	/6	WIDE-GRIP PULLUP	/10	/8	/8	/6
CORKSCREW	/10	/10	/10	/10	CABLE PARALLEL	/10	/10	/10	/10
PLANK	30–45 sec	30–45 sec	30–45 sec	30–45 sec	SIDE PLANK + REACH	30–45 sec	30–45 sec	30–45 sec	30–45 sec

EXERCISE	1	2	3	4	EXERCISE	1	2	3	4
WORKOUT A2					WORKOUT B2				
HIGH PULL	/3	/3	/3	/3	HANG POWER CLEAN	/3	/3	/3	/3
1-LEG SQUAT	/10	/8	/8	/6	SEATED GOOD MORN	/10	/8	/8	/6
PUSHUP	/10	/8	/8	/6	HORIZ SIDE-TO-SIDE PULLUP	/10	/8	/8	/6
CABLE PRESS	/10	/8	/8	/6	LAT PLDWN	/10	/8	/8	/6
WOOD CHOP KNEE	/10	/10	/10	/10	MED BALL OVER SHOULDER	/10	/10	/10	/10
POST BRIDGE	30–45 sec	30–45 sec	30–45 sec	30–45 sec	CORE ROW	30–45 sec	30–45 sec	30–45 sec	30–45 sec

STRENGTH TRAINING

The purpose of this strength-training program is obviously to develop as much muscular strength as possible. Unlike the hypertrophy program, this program is characterized by lower work volumes and much higher intensities (loads). There is still an alternating pattern every 3 weeks but the changes in volumes and loads are not all that significant. The results for this particular training program will be greater muscular strength as assessed by 1- to 5-repetition maximums. The sample programs found in this chapter will highlight both full-body and push-pull routines.

As with the hypertrophy program, I suggest shifting back to the total fitness program after completing the 12-week strength-training program. After completing the next 12 weeks of total fitness training, you can return to the strength program for another 12 weeks.

Average training volumes per exercise

Weeks 1 to 3 = 24

Weeks 4 to 6 = 15

Weeks 7 to 9 = 20

Weeks 10 to 12 = 11

Rest periods

Explosive Exercises = 90 seconds to 2 minutes

1 to 6 reps = 90 seconds to 2 minutes

8 to 12 reps = 60 seconds

Complexing allowed = YES

Unloading recommendations = At least one to two sessions every 6 weeks

SAMPLE 3-DAY FULL-BODY WORKOUT FOR STRENGTH TRAINING (WEEKS 10–12)

WEEK 10

MOVEMENT	EXERCISE	1	2	3	4	
	WORKOUT A					
EXPLOSIVE	HANG POWER CLEAN	/3	/3	/3	/3	
KNEE DOMINANT	FRONT SQUAT	/5	/3	/2	/1	
HIP DOMINANT	1-LEG ROM DEADLIFT	/5	/3	/2	/1	
HORIZONTAL PUSH	BENCH PRESS	/5	/3	/2	/1	
HORIZONTAL PULL	DB ROW	/5	/3	/2	/1	
VERTICAL PUSH	PUSH PRESS	/5	/3	/2	/1	
VERTICAL PULL	1-ARM LAT PLDWN	/5	/3	/2	/1	
ROTATIONAL	SEATED RUSS TWIST	/8	/8	/8	/8	
BRIDGING	PLANK ELBOW TO KNEE	30–45 sec	30–45 sec	30–45 sec	30–45 sec	

WEEK 11

MOVEMENT	EXERCISE	1	2	3	4	
	WORKOUT B					
EXPLOSIVE	MUSCLE SNATCH	/3	/3	/3	/3	
KNEE DOMINANT	1-LEG SQUAT	/5	/3	/2	/1	
HIP DOMINANT	ROM DEADLIFT	/5	/3	/2	/1	
HORIZONTAL PUSH	DB 1-ARM ON BALL	/5	/3	/2	/1	
HORIZONTAL PULL	CABLE FACE PULL	/5	/3	/2	/1	
VERTICAL PUSH	DB SPLIT JERK	/5	/3	/2	/1	
VERTICAL PULL	CHINUP	/5	/3	/2	/1	
ROTATIONAL	PARALLEL SWING	/8	/8	/8	/8	
BRIDGING	DYNAMIC PLANK	30–45 sec	30–45 sec	30–45 sec	30–45 sec	

WEEK 12

MOVEMENT	EXERCISE	1	2	3	4	
	WORKOUT A					
EXPLOSIVE	DB SNATCH	/3	/3	/3	/3	
KNEE DOMINANT	OVRHD SQUAT	/5	/3	/2	/1	
HIP DOMINANT	1-LEG BACK EXT	/5	/3	/2	/1	
HORIZONTAL PUSH	INCLINE BENCH PRESS	/5	/3	/2	/1	
HORIZONTAL PULL	DB ROW	/5	/3	/2	/1	
VERTICAL PUSH	PUSH JERK	/5	/3	/2	/1	
VERTICAL PULL	SIDE-TO-SIDE PULLUP	/5	/3	/2	/1	
ROTATIONAL	REV WOOD CHOP	/8	/8	/8	/8	
BRIDGING	SUPINE BRIDGE	30–45 sec	30–45 sec	30–45 sec	30–45 sec	

EXERCISE	1	2	3	4	EXERCISE	1	2	3	4
WORKOUT B					**WORKOUT A**				
HANG JUMP SHRUG	/3	/3	/3	/3	SNATCH PULL	/3	/3	/3	/3
DROP LUNGE	/5	/3	/2	/1	SPLIT SQUAT	/5	/3	/2	/1
GOOD MORN	/5	/3	/2	/1	1-LEG BACK EXT	/5	/3	/2	/1
DB INCLINE BENCH PRESS	/5	/3	/2	/1	REV-GRIP BENCH PRESS	/5	/3	/2	/1
HORIZ PULLUP	/5	/3	/2	/1	1-ARM CABLE ROW	/5	/3	/2	/1
SUPPORTED DB 1-ARM PRESS	/5	/3	/2	/1	PUSH JERK	/5	/3	/2	/1
WIDE-GRIP PULLUP	/5	/3	/2	/1	SIDE-TO-SIDE PULLUP	/5	/3	/2	/1
CORKSCREW	/8	/8	/8	/8	WOOD CHOP	/8	/8	/8	/8
PLANK	30–45 sec	30–45 sec	30–45 sec	30–45 sec	PLANK WALKUP	30–45 sec	30–45 sec	30–45 sec	30–45 sec

EXERCISE	1	2	3	4	EXERCISE	1	2	3	4
WORKOUT A					**WORKOUT B**				
HANG POWER SNATCH	/3	/3	/3	/3	DB HANG POWER CLEAN	/3	/3	/3	/3
BACK SQUAT	/5	/3	/2	/1	BULG SPLIT SQUAT	/5	/3	/2	/1
1-LEG GOOD MORN	/5	/3	/2	/1	ROM DEADLIFT	/5	/3	/2	/1
BENCH PRESS	/5	/3	/2	/1	DB INCLINE ON BALL	/5	/3	/2	/1
DB ROW + TWIST	/5	/3	/2	/1	CABLE ROW TO NECK	/5	/3	/2	/1
PUSH PRESS	/5	/3	/2	/1	DB PUSH JERK	/5	/3	/2	/1
1-ARM PLDWN	/5	/3	/2	/1	CHINUP	/5	/3	/2	/1
SWISS BALL WT ROLL	/8	/8	/8	/8	BB TORQUE	/8	/8	/8	/8
SIDE PLANK	30–45 sec	30–45 sec	30–45 sec	30–45 sec	PLANK W/ WT TRANS	30–45 sec	30–45 sec	30–45 sec	30–45 sec

EXERCISE	1	2	3	4	EXERCISE	1	2	3	4
WORKOUT B					**WORKOUT A**				
CLEAN PULL	/3	/3	/3	/3	POWER CLEAN	/3	/3	/3	/3
STEPUP	/5	/3	/2	/1	SPLIT SQUAT	/5	/3	/2	/1
SEATED GOOD MORN	/5	/3	/2	/1	1-LEG ROM DEADLIFT	/5	/3	/2	/1
SIDE-TO-SIDE PUSHUP	/5	/3	/2	/1	DIP	/5	/3	/2	/1
CABLE ROW	/5	/3	/2	/1	1-ARM CABLE ROW TO NECK	/5	/3	/2	/1
DB PUSH PRESS	/5	/3	/2	/1	SPLIT JERK	/5	/3	/2	/1
MIXED-GRIP PULLUP	/5	/3	/2	/1	SIDE-TO-SIDE PULLUP	/5	/3	/2	/1
WOOD CHOP KNEE	/8	/8	/8	/8	SEATED RUSS TWIST	/8	/8	/8	/8
SIDE PLANK REACH	30–45 sec	30–45 sec	30–45 sec	30–45 sec	PLANK WALKUP	30–45 sec	30–45 sec	30–45 sec	30–45 sec

SAMPLE 4-DAY PUSH-PULL WORKOUT FOR STRENGTH TRAINING (WEEKS 4–6)

WEEK 4

MOVEMENT	EXERCISE	1	2	3	4	EXERCISE	1	2	3	4
	WORKOUT A1					WORKOUT B1				
EXPLOSIVE	CLEAN PULL	/3	/3	/3	/3	MUSCLE SNATCH	/3	/3	/3	/3
HIP/KNEE DOMINANT	FRONT SQUAT	/6	/4	/3	/2	1-LEG ROM DEADLIFT	/6	/4	/3	/2
HORIZONTAL PUSH/PULL	DB BENCH PRESS	/6	/4	/3	/2	CABLE FACE PULL	/6	/4	/3	/2
VERTICAL PUSH/PULL	PUSH PRESS	/6	/4	/3	/2	1-ARM PLDWN	/6	/4	/3	/2
ROTATIONAL	WOOD CHOP	/8	/8	/8	/8	SEATED RUSS TWIST	/8	/8	/8	/8
BRIDGING	PLANK	30–45 sec	30–45 sec	30–45 sec	30–45 sec	SIDE PLANK + REACH	30–45 sec	30–45 sec	30–45 sec	30–45 sec

WEEK 5

MOVEMENT	EXERCISE	1	2	3	4	EXERCISE	1	2	3	4
	WORKOUT A1					WORKOUT B1				
EXPLOSIVE	DB SNATCH	/3	/3	/3	/3	HANG POWER CLEAN	/3	/3	/3	/3
HIP/KNEE DOMINANT	SPLIT SQUAT	/6	/4	/3	/2	1-LEG BACK EXT	/6	/4	/3	/2
HORIZONTAL PUSH/PULL	SIDE-TO-SIDE PUSHUP	/6	/4	/3	/2	HORIZ PULLUP	/6	/4	/3	/2
VERTICAL PUSH/PULL	JACKKNIFE PUSHUP	/6	/4	/3	/2	SIDE-TO-SIDE PULLUP	/6	/4	/3	/2
ROTATIONAL	CABLE PUSH-PULL ROT	/8	/8	/8	/8	MED BALL 1-2-3	/8	/8	/8	/8
BRIDGING	SIDE PLANK	30–45 sec	30–45 sec	30–45 sec	30–45 sec	DYNAMIC PLANK	30–45 sec	30–45 sec	30–45 sec	30–45 sec

WEEK 6

MOVEMENT	EXERCISE	1	2	3	4	EXERCISE	1	2	3	4
	WORKOUT A1					WORKOUT B1				
EXPLOSIVE	CLEAN PULL	/3	/3	/3	/3	SNATCH PULL	/3	/3	/3	/3
HIP/KNEE DOMINANT	BACK SQUAT	/6	/4	/3	/2	1-LEG GOOD MORN	/6	/4	/3	/2
HORIZONTAL PUSH/PULL	DB INCLINE BENCH PRESS	/6	/4	/3	/2	BENT-OVR ROW	/6	/4	/3	/2
VERTICAL PUSH/PULL	SPLIT JERK	/6	/4	/3	/2	1-ARM PLDWN	/6	/4	/3	/2
ROTATIONAL	SWISS BALL WT ROLL	/8	/8	/8	/8	BB TORQUE	/8	/8	/8	/8
BRIDGING	PLANK W/ ELBOW TO KNEE	30–45 sec	30–45 sec	30–45 sec	30–45 sec	PLANK W/ WT TRANS	30–45 sec	30–45 sec	30–45 sec	30–45 sec

EXERCISE	1	2	3	4	EXERCISE	1	2	3	4
WORKOUT A2					**WORKOUT B2**				
DB HANG CLEAN	/3	/3	/3	/3	NARROW-GRIP HANG SNATCH	/3	/3	/3	/3
STEPUP	/6	/4	/3	/2	ROM DEADLIFT	/6	/4	/3	/2
CLOSE-GRIP BENCH PRESS	/6	/4	/3	/2	DB ROW + TWIST	/6	/4	/3	/2
SUPPORTED DB 1-ARM PRESS	/6	/4	/3	/2	CHINUP	/6	/4	/3	/2
WINDSHIELD WIPER	/8	/8	/8	/8	REV WOOD CHOP KNEE	/8	/8	/8	/8
PLANK WALKUP	30–45 sec	30–45 sec	30–45 sec	30–45 sec	2-PT PLANK	30–45 sec	30–45 sec	30–45 sec	30–45 sec

EXERCISE	1	2	3	4	EXERCISE	1	2	3	4
WORKOUT A2					**WORKOUT B2**				
HANG JUMP SHRUG	/3	/3	/3	/3	CLEAN PULL	/3	/3	/3	/3
BULG SPLIT SQUAT	/6	/4	/3	/2	GOOD MORN	/6	/4	/3	/2
REV-GRIP BENCH PRESS	/6	/4	/3	/2	1-ARM CABLE ROW	/6	/4	/3	/2
DB PUSH PRESS	/6	/4	/3	/2	WIDE-GRIP PULLUP	/6	/4	/3	/2
CORKSCREW	/8	/8	/8	/8	CABLE PARALLEL	/8	/8	/8	/8
PLANK	30–45 sec	30–45 sec	30–45 sec	30–45 sec	SIDE PLANK + REACH	30–45 sec	30–45 sec	30–45 sec	30–45 sec

EXERCISE	1	2	3	4	EXERCISE	1	2	3	4
WORKOUT A2					**WORKOUT B2**				
HIGH PULL	/3	/3	/3	/3	HANG POWER CLEAN	/3	/3	/3	/3
1-LEG SQUAT	/6	/4	/3	/2	SEATED GOOD MORN	/6	/4	/3	/2
PUSHUP	/6	/4	/3	/2	HORIZ SIDE-TO-SIDE PULLUP	/6	/4	/3	/2
CABLE PRESS	/6	/4	/3	/2	LAT PLDWN	/6	/4	/3	/2
WOOD CHOP KNEE	/8	/8	/8	/8	MED BALL OVER SHOULDER	/8	/8	/8	/8
POST. BRIDGE	30–45 sec	30–45 sec	30–45 sec	30–45 sec	CORE ROW	30–45 sec	30–45 sec	30–45 sec	30–45 sec

PART 5

POWER TRAINING EXTRAS

POWER TRAINING NUTRITION

Like the fitness industry, the nutrition world has an abundance of "experts" and "gurus," each touting his or her plan as the best in the business. I have heard just about all the nutrition experts and have read all of the "new and improved" eating plans at our disposal these days. My friend Alwyn Cosgrove has a great description for most of these programs—he calls them "hot dog programs." On the surface these programs are just like hot dogs: They are very popular and they seem great, but when you start to dissect them and take a good look at what's inside, you realize that you really don't want anything to do with them. I recently had the opportunity to meet and discuss nutrition with Mike Roussell, a doctoral student in nutrition at Pennsylvania State University and one of the sharpest young minds in the nutrition world. Mike is also the author of Your Naked Nutrition Guide: Nutrition Stripped to the Essentials. *In his book, Mike has put together one of the soundest eating guides I have come across, so of course I was thrilled when he agreed to write the nutrition chapter you are about to read here.*

As you read through this book, you will notice that Robert dos Remedios has an effective, no-nonsense, no-gimmicks approach to training. The nutritional strategies I am going to outline in this chapter mirror this sentiment. The world of nutrition, like the world of training, is full of gimmicks. However, the core message is always the most important, which is why I call my approach Naked Nutrition. All the gimmicks and false promises have been stripped away, leaving practical, effective, simple nutrition strategies you can apply to your life and training schedule to maximize the effectiveness of the programs outlined in this book.

THE BIG LIE

Before we delve into the basics of Naked Nutrition, it is important to step back and briefly discuss goal setting and the importance of having a long-term plan. The nutrition world is full of promises of extreme fat loss and/or muscle growth that occurs in a matter of weeks. This is what I call "The Big Lie" because, unfortunately, these promises are, more often than not, empty. People bounce from quick fix to quick fix before realizing that months, if not years, have gone by and no noticeable progress has been made. This is why long-term planning is so important. By mapping out what you want to achieve with your body over the next year, your chances of achieving those changes increase exponentially. Grab a pen and write down exactly what you want to be able to do and what you want to look like in 1 year. How strong will you be? How lean will you be? The more specific the better.

Unfortunately, progress—whether it is fat loss or muscle growth—does not happen in a linear fashion week in and week out. Common estimates for fat loss are 1 to 2 pounds per week, while estimates for muscle growth are 1 to 3 pounds per month. On a weekly basis, you may not see this kind of progress, but when you look at your training over the course of several months, it often averages out to this. Expecting consistent linear progress often leaves people frustrated and tempted to try the newest "secret" in training. I call this "falling off the wagon," and it can be avoided by implementing solid long-term planning and by using multiple methods of measurement.

The scale is the most common method people use to gauge their progress. However, the scale does not tell you whether you are gaining or losing fat or muscle. For example, if over the course of 2 weeks you lost 1 pound of fat but gained 1 pound of muscle, the scale would read the same as it did at the beginning of those 2 weeks. This can be discouraging because it seems as if you have not made any progress. The real story is that the opposite is true. You have, in fact, made remarkable progress. This is why you need multiple methods of measurement—so that you get the most accurate depiction of your progress. Here is how I recommend you track your progress.

1. **Daily weights.** Record your weight every morning upon waking. While your weight can fluctuate on a daily basis over the course of days and weeks, you will get an accurate read on your progress.

2. **Girth measurements.** Measure the circumference of your neck, shoulders, chest, arms, waist, thighs, and calves every 2 to 3 weeks.

3. **Body fat measurements.** Measure your body fat by using body fat calipers every 2 to 3 weeks. Don't just record your body fat, but also record the actual caliper measurements as these will give you insight into if you are gaining or losing body fat in particular areas of your body.

4. **Strength measures.** Keep an accurate record of all your lifts and weights in the gym. Strength gains are more often than not accompanied by muscle gains.

NEW FOOD GROUPS FOR THE 21ST CENTURY

During the mid-1950s, the USDA unleashed on the world the four basic food groups: Dairy, Meat, Fruits and Vegetables, and Grains. Nutrition was simple. Simply eat foods from these four groups at each of your three "square" meals every day. While these categorizations of foods and meal times worked fine for the average person, they don't if you are following the Power Training program. In this chapter, you will be introduced to the Six Pillars of Nutrition and your new rules for eating. The Six Pillars of Nutrition are guided by the science of nutrient timing, which is the concept that your body uses certain nutrients better at different times of the day, and the *new* food groups, which are a slight twist on the four old basics. The new food groups separate foods into protein, fats, fruits and vegetables, and starches. These categories will be explained in the following pages as part of the Six Pillars of Nutrition.

Six Pillars of Nutrition

1. Eat five or six times a day.

2. Limit your consumption of sugars and processed foods.

3. Eat fruits and vegetables throughout the day.

4. Drink more water and cut out calorie-containing beverages (beer, soda, and so forth).

5. Focus on consuming lean proteins throughout the day.

6. Save starch-containing foods until after a workout or for breakfast.

EAT FIVE OR SIX TIMES A DAY

As an active person following the training routines and principles outlined in this book, you are going to need more calories than the average person. You also can't eat on the same schedule as an average person. In order to build muscle and strength and keep your metabolism functioning optimally, you are going to need to consume a substantial amount of calories. To do this effectively, the traditional three square meals a day isn't going to cut it. Instead, you will need to eat twice as often (five or six times a day), consuming nutrient-rich meals every 2 to 3 hours. By eating this way, you will be constantly feeding your body the nutrients it needs to recover from workouts, build muscle, control blood sugar, and optimize performance. The larger you are, the more calories you need and the more meals you will need to consume. For example, if you weigh between 150 and 200 pounds, five or six meals will do. However, if you weigh 200 to 250 pounds, then you will need to consume six or seven meals. Adjusting the number of meals you consume in relation to the total number of calories you consume will allow you to continue eating reasonable portion sizes without overloading your body with too many calories at once.

LIMIT YOUR CONSUMPTION OF SUGARS AND PROCESSED FOODS

If you could only implement one change in your nutritional plan, it should be to limit/eliminate your consumption of sugars and processed foods. By doing this, you will remove sugary calorie-containing beverages like artificially sweetened iced tea, soda, and those $5 lattés. Abiding by this pillar will also ensure that you're no longer eating other calorie-dense, nutrient-poor foods such as chips, white bread, high-fat processed meats, cookies, and french fries (to name a few). Remember, it is not a good thing if someone asks you about the orange-colored foods you eat and you respond with "cheese curls" and not carrots or sweet potatoes. By cutting out processed food, you will also be forced to eat fresh, healthy, nutrient-rich foods such as fruits, vegetables, and lean proteins. This is a phenomenon known as dietary displacement. Not only is consuming large amounts of sugar-filled processed foods unhealthy, but also by consuming those calories you prevent yourself from consuming wholesome unprocessed foods that will allow you to reduce your body fat, increase your strength, and build muscle—not to mention greatly improve your health.

EAT FRUITS AND VEGETABLES THROUGHOUT THE DAY

It is unfortunate that I was involved in the area of high-performance nutrition for several years before fully grasping the importance of consuming large amounts of fruits and vegetables. Bodybuilders and athletes are often portrayed in magazines eating plates full of chicken breast and plain brown rice, not plates full of fruits and vegetables. You should eat more fruits and vegetables than any of the other *new* food groups. What makes fruits and vegetables such a valuable piece of your nutritional arsenal is that they are loaded with vitamins, minerals, phytochemicals, and fiber. Plus their sheer bulk allows you to maintain a high level of satiety or fullness throughout the day while controlling your blood sugar and insulin levels.

If you were to ask most people what the most powerful hormone in the body is for building muscle, most would answer with testosterone. In fact, the correct answer to what is the body's most powerful promoter of protein synthesis is insulin. To control insulin is to control your body composition. The best part about insulin, unlike testosterone, is that you can completely control insulin through diet.

Insulin is a hormone released from your pancreas in response to increases in sugar and amino acid levels in your blood. Its main job is to get sugar and amino acids out of the bloodstream and into various tissues in the body (e.g., muscle and fat tissue). Insulin's action can be good or bad depending on the time of day and your goals. The beneficial side of insulin is that during and after exercise, it will preferentially shuttle sugar and amino acids to your muscle, allowing for increased growth and recovery. Aside from the anabolic effects of shuttling nutrients into muscles, insulin also has a direct effect on promoting protein synthesis, speeding the rate at which your body builds muscle.

The downside of insulin is that it inhibits fat cells from releasing stored fat (i.e., stops fat burning). Current research suggests that increases in blood sugar levels and insulin during and directly after exercise do not inhibit fat loss. However, throughout the rest of the day it is prudent to control insulin levels. The Six Pillars of Nutrition emphasize starchy carbohydrates in the morning and during or following workouts to maximize the benefits of insulin while minimizing its detrimental effects through eating lower-impact carbohydrates such as fruits and vegetables throughout the rest of the day.

DRINK MORE WATER AND CUT OUT CALORIE-CONTAINING BEVERAGES

Water is the best performance-enhancing "drug" out there. Studies have shown that maintaining a proper level of hydration before, during, and after exercise helps maintain performance, lower exercising heart rate, reduce heat stress, and prevent drops in strength due to dehydration. If you are serious about performing at the highest level possible, you need to make sure that you are properly hydrated.

A good place to start is drinking a glass of water with each meal, one upon waking up, and one just before bed. Using these guidelines, you will be drinking seven to eight glasses a day easily.

Two quick ways to ensure you are properly hydrated are the following:

• Have two completely clear urinations each day.

• Never allow yourself to get thirsty. If you find yourself thirsty, you are already on your way to becoming dehydrated.

I must add one note of caution: *Do not overhydrate.* Greatly overconsuming water can lead to electrolyte imbalances in your body. This will lead to a decrease in performance or, worse yet, a trip to the hospital.

FOCUS ON CONSUMING LEAN PROTEINS THROUGHOUT THE DAY

There has been an anti-protein movement among many nutritionists and dietitians where claims are made such as "You only need 0.8 gram of protein per kilogram of body weight" and "If you consume excess protein, your body will excrete the extra nitrogen and you'll just have expensive urine." But these claims are made when people just think of protein and amino acids as the building blocks of muscle. There is actually research that suggests athletes who train with weights may need *less* protein than those who do not.

This seems to be due to the body's adaptation and more efficient use of protein.

However, to eat only protein because its amino acids serve as the building blocks of muscle would be doing this macronutrient a great disservice. Consuming lean proteins throughout the day has other very important benefits.

Decreased insulin response. Increasing your protein consumption will mean that you will have to displace other foods from your diet. This displacement normally comes at the expense of carbohydrates, and protein can be a beneficial replacement because it stimulates much less insulin than carbohydrates. If you remember, controlling insulin is a very important part of the Naked Nutrition approach.

Increased thermic effect of food. When you eat food, it "costs" your body energy to break down, digest, and turn it into an energy source it can use. This caloric cost is called the thermic effect of food (TEF). Protein has a higher TEF than either carbohydrate or fat. This added TEF will help boost your metabolism—always a good thing.

Increased protein synthesis. In addition to being the building blocks of muscle, certain amino acids, such as leucine, can turn on and regulate genes in your body associated with protein synthesis and muscle growth.

SAVE STARCH-CONTAINING FOODS UNTIL AFTER A WORKOUT OR FOR BREAKFAST

Starchy carbohydrates are food such as grains, potatoes, corn, or sugar. When these foods are eaten, they cause a relatively fast increase in blood sugar levels. Because these carbohydrates are easily consumed in larger quantities, they can also stimulate insulin to a greater degree than fruits and vegetables. Starchy carbohydrates are generally carbohydrates that have a high to medium glycemic index rating. The glycemic index is a number given to carbohydrates, on a scale of 1 to 100, rating them on how quickly the sugars from the carbohydrates enter the bloodstream. The faster sugars enter your system, the higher the glycemic index and the faster your blood sugar levels will go up. Keeping blood sugar levels under control and at a consistent level has been a theme throughout this chapter, but there are certain times when increases in blood sugar levels and insulin are beneficial—in the morning and during your workouts are two of these times.

First let's look at the benefits of consuming starchy, whole-grain carbohydrates for breakfast.

Your liver glycogen levels are low in the morning. Your body's metabolic brain is the liver. The liver is the hub for almost all things metabolically related. One of the most important actions the liver has as the metabolic brain is controlling blood sugar levels when carbohydrates are not being eaten. To do this the liver has the capability to store a moderate amount of carbohydrates in an easily accessible form known as glycogen. When organs and various tissues in the body (such as brain and muscle) take sugar from the bloodstream, the liver releases its stored glycogen to fill the void. While you are sleeping, liver glycogen is a major source of fuel for the body, since most of us don't eat in our sleep. This means that when you wake up in the morning, your liver glycogen levels are at an all-time low. Consuming starchy carbohydrates will quickly refill your liver's glycogen stores. Some people abstain from starchy grains early in the morning out of fear that they will be stored as body fat. Yet these carbohydrates won't be stored as fat. Instead, they will be used to refill the liver's glycogen stores as well as to fuel your morning activities.

Early-morning carbohydrates create a beneficial hormonal environment. The levels of various hormones in your body fluctuate throughout the day through what is known as a diurnal rhythm, a rhythm based on the day/night cycle. Hormones, such as testosterone and cortisol, which follow this diurnal rhythm, are higher in the morning and lower later in the day. Cortisol is an important hormone because your body needs it to cope with stress. However it can be a double-edged sword as some of cortisol's other actions include breaking down muscle and stimulating fat storage. Certain levels of cortisol are needed for your body to function properly, but excess levels can be detrimental. Insulin is a hormone that counteracts cortisol. By consuming starches in the morning when your cortisol level is at its highest, you can stimulate the release of insulin, which can help blunt and reduce cortisol's effect. This puts your body in a hormonal environment that is conducive to muscle growth, not muscle loss.

WORKOUT NUTRITION

One of the problems with exercise, and weight training in particular, is that it doesn't build muscle. In fact, it breaks muscle down. Weight training is a destructive process. It is the reforming and rebuilding of more muscle tissue and stronger muscles that makes hitting the iron three or four times a week worthwhile. Proper nutrition is important throughout the day, but during the workout and post-workout periods, certain nutritional interventions can have an incredible effect on your recovery, growth, and performance. Rules that are extremely important to follow in regards to workout nutrition are (1) liquid calories and (2) carbohydrates and protein.

Let's look at these two in more detail.

Liquid calories. The Naked Nutrition plan for Power Training is based around consuming fresh whole foods. However, during your workout there is a benefit to surpassing the whole food option and opting for liquid calories. Digesting whole foods requires a lot of mechanical work and effort from your body. In order for this mechanical work to occur, your body needs to send blood to your stomach so that fuel and oxygen can be given to the hard-working tissues. Unfortunately, if the blood is going to your stomach, then it can't go to your muscles. Consuming liquid calories allows for as little mechanical digestion as possible, so the nutrients can get into your system and the blood to your muscles. Liquid calories get into your system very quickly.

Another benefit of consuming liquid calories is that they can be easily consumed slowly over a long period of time. It is no problem to sip on a workout drink throughout your 60-minute workout, but trying to eat chicken breasts and brown rice between sets of dumbbell snatches is a whole different story!

Carbohydrates and protein. For years, workout nutrition has been associated with carbohydrates. Whether it is Gatorade or orange juice, active people have been fueling their workouts with carbohydrates. Carbohydrate consumption before, during, and after your workouts is very important as these carbohydrates will help blunt cortisol release, stimulate insulin release, and replenish your muscle glycogen stores so that your body is ready to go for its next training session.

While consuming liquid carbohydrates is better than just drinking water, new sports nutrition research consistently shows that adding a small amount of protein or amino acids (the molecules that make up protein) to your workout drink will make a huge difference in your progress. A recent study examined the effects of a carbohydrate workout drink verses a carbohydrates + amino acid drink over the course of a 12-week training period. At the end of 12 weeks, both groups lost approximately 4 pounds of body fat. However, the carbohydrates + amino acid group gained 5 pounds more muscle (for a total of more than 9 pounds) than the carbohydrate group.

The addition of protein to your previously carbohydrate-only drink will reduce muscle breakdown, lower cortisol, and increase insulin more than a carbohydrate-only drink. Earlier I mentioned that insulin control is extremely important throughout the day, and it is, but during and after your workout it is very important to manipulate your nutrition so that your body releases insulin for growth and recovery. Insulin is a potent stimulator of muscle growth.

WORKOUT PRESCRIPTION

Your workout nutrition should begin 20 minutes before you actually start your workout. This means that while driving to the gym or while you are getting dressed in the locker room, you should be sipping on your workout shake. Depending on your body size, I recommend 50 to 60 grams of sugar (preferably dextrose and/or maltodextrose) along with 15 to 25 grams of protein. Why dextrose and maltodextrose? Dextose is another word for glucose. Glucose is the most basic form of sugar. In its most basic form, sugar gets absorbed by your body and put to work fueling your workout and recovery very quickly. Maltodextrose is a chain of dextrose molecules strung together. It also provides readily available fuel to your body. Most commercial workout shakes will include dextrose and/or maltodextrose. I use this prescription for calorie intakes ranging from 2,000 to 3,500 calories. If you are consuming caloric amounts outside these ranges, you will need to adjust the recommendations either up or down. You can combine a liquid carbohydrate drink with a protein powder or buy a workout shake containing a mixture of protein and carbohydrates. The premixed powders are typically more expensive, but they are extremely convenient. Regardless of which you pick, choose a product that contains either whey protein isolate or whey protein hydrolysate. Whey protein isolate is a very pure form of whey protein. It tastes better than whey protein concentrates and usually has all the lactose removed (which is good for those who are lactose intolerant). Whey protein hydrolysate is similar to whey protein isolate in purity, but it is processed one step further and the protein chains are chopped up into smaller fragments. These smaller fragments require little to no mechanical or chemical digestion and get into your body extremely fast.

If you have any of your shake left once you finish your workout, drink it. Be prepared to eat again 45 to 60 minutes after you finish off your shake. Eating again soon after your workout is important to keep your body in an anabolic (muscle-building) environment and to keep your blood sugar at a moderate level. Sometimes 45 to 60 minutes after consuming a workout shake like the one described above, your blood sugar levels can drop too low, which will make you feel lousy and potentially hinder recovery.

PUTTING TOGETHER MEAL PLANS BY FOCUSING ON FOOD CHOICES

One of the most important concepts to grasp in this chapter outside the Six Pillars is that you do *not* need to count calories. Counting calories for most people is a waste of time. Plus who has the time? Counting the caloric value of every piece of food that crosses your lips is a full-time job! Instead, you really only need to focus on making consistently proper food choices. The Six Pillars of Nutrition were designed so that when implemented, you wouldn't need to count calories to get results. By focusing on eating certain types of foods at certain times throughout the day, you will be able to build a strong and lean body without the unnecessary hassle of counting calories.

The most common problem that I find with people and their nutrition is lack of compliance (the second is undereating). If you have a great plan but don't follow it, you might as well have had a terrible plan. I learned from well-known nutritionist John Berardi, PhD, the importance of tracking how well you stick to your meal plan. Dr. Berardi calls it the 90 percent rule. This means that you need to follow your meal plan at least 90 percent of the time before you can determine whether it is working. If you don't follow your plan 90 percent of the time, then you aren't really following your plan now, are you? The 90 percent rule also allows you to eat whatever you want 10 percent of the time. So if you are craving pizza, ice cream, or a rack of ribs from your favorite rib joint, that's fine as long as you follow your plan 90 percent of the time.

WHERE TO START

One strategy that is guaranteed to fail you is what I call "nutritional freestyling." Nutritional freestyling is not thinking about what you are going to eat until it is time to eat. This never works because it involves too much thinking about food on the spot and it often puts you in a position where you will make poor food choices. Instead, you need a plan. By taking the time to sit down on Sunday afternoon, plan out and prepare your meals for the week, you will take the *thinking* out of eating during the week. You will have a much easier time eating properly during the week

when your life gets busy because you won't have to think about what to eat and where to get it as your food will be right there prepared for you.

The real key to nutritional success is finding a plan that you can really implement and adopt as part of your lifestyle. To make sure your nutrition changes stick, it is important to make gradual changes. If you are currently only eating two to three meals a day and rarely allow a vegetable to cross your lips, jumping into six strict meals per day and measuring out all your foods will probably be too much of a shock to your system. Instead, gradually increase your meal frequency over the course of 3 to 6 weeks so that by the end, you are eating five to six meals a day. At the same time, start to incorporate each of the Six Pillars of Nutrition into your daily eating. Easing yourself into the Naked Nutrition style of eating will ensure that you adopt these habits as part of your everyday life— and not just as a transient diet.

When you first start out, don't even worry about the amounts of foods you are eating—just get the selection down. Here is an example of what a typical meal plan might look like. This meal plan contains approximately 3,000 calories.

Training Day Meal Plan 1

Meal 1

6 egg whites and 1 whole egg, scrambled

1 ounce lean turkey ham

¼ cup diced onions and ¼ cup diced peppers

1 cup oatmeal (dry measure)

Meal 2

2 scoops protein powder (milk protein blend,
such as Metabolic Drive from Biotest) with 8
ounces water

1 ounce almonds

1 medium apple

Meal 3

5 cups lettuce or spinach

10 cherry tomatoes

¾ cup sliced cucumbers

¼ cup feta cheese

6 ounces roasted chicken (raw weight)

1 tablespoon olive oil

Meal 4: Workout Shake

50–60 grams carbohydrates

15–25 grams whey protein isolate or
hydrosylate

Meal 5

6 ounces grilled pork loin (raw weight)

2 grilled pineapple slices

4 cups spinach with olive oil (2 teaspoons)

1¾ cups brown rice (cooked measure)

Meal 6

1 cup cottage cheese

½ cup blueberries

1 ounce slivered almonds

Notice how the meal plan is laid out so that it follows the Six Pillars of Nutrition. Each meal contains protein and fruits/vegetables. The starchy carbohydrates are found in Meal 1 (oatmeal) and Meals 4 (workout) and 5 (brown rice) during or following the workout. Beverages containing empty calories and processed foods have all been eliminated. The meal plan is based around eating solid foods except for during the workout, when liquid nutrition is essential, and in Meal 2. A protein shake is used as the protein source in Meal 2 more for convenience than anything else. Most people have busy lives and can't always find the time during the work day to sit down and eat a salad. In situations like that a protein shake, a piece of fruit, and some nuts is a great, portable, and versatile meal option. If you are really in a bind then a protein bar would be your next best choice. Most protein bars contain large amounts of sugar so be careful and read the labels. That is why I don't normally recommend protein bars as dietary staples, but rather as nutritional backups. Another strategy for those with busy lives is to eat the same thing twice in one day. When you are eating five or six times a day, food preparation becomes more involved than when you were eating the traditional "three square meals." Eating the same meal twice can greatly reduce meal preparation as you can just make twice as much of one item. This works with both whole food meals and shakes—for shakes just make sure your blender is big enough (see the nonworkout day meal plan for an example of this).

Here are some more sample meal plans you can use.

Training Day Meal Plan 2 (3,000 calories)

Meal 1

Breakfast on the Go Shake

1½ scoops protein powder

2 cup frozen mixed berries

2 tablespoons chopped walnuts

½ cup rolled oats (dry measure)

*Add water, ice cubes, and blend together.

Meal 2

1 cup cottage cheese

1 tablespoon peanut butter

½ scoop chocolate protein powder (for flavor and added protein)

1 sliced banana

*Mix all together in a bowl.

Meal 3

8 ounces grilled flank steak (rubbed with chili powder, garlic, salt, and pepper)

3 cups broccoli florets

½ tablespoon olive oil

Meal 4: Workout Shake

50–60 grams carbohydrates

15–25 grams whey protein isolate or hydrosylate

Meal 5

5 ounces oven-roasted trout with cilantro, lemon, and garlic

2½ cups mashed sweet potatoes

Meal 6

Chicken Salad

¾ cup diced chicken breast

1 tablespoon light canola mayonnaise

1 cup grapes

1 diced celery stalk

½ cup red onion

2 tablespoons chopped walnuts

Salt and pepper to taste

*Eat over 3 cups of romaine lettuce.

For Nonworkout Days (2,500 calories)

On nonworkout days you will naturally eat fewer calories because you won't have a workout shake and you will be eating fewer starches. This drop in calories is a simplified version of calorie cycling and is effective at keeping additional fat gain at bay.

Meal 1

3 slices whole wheat toast

4 egg white + 1 whole egg omelet

¼ cup reduced-fat mozzarella

¾ cup chopped tomatoes

½ lean Italian chicken sausage

Meal 2

1½ scoops chocolate protein powder

1 banana

¼ cup shredded unsweetened coconut

2 tablespoons flaxmeal

4 ice cubes

*Add water and blend to desired consistency.

Meal 3

4 cups spinach

4 ounces grilled chicken breast (raw weight)

¼ cup crumbled blue cheese

1 medium apple, diced

10 cherry tomatoes

Meal 4

1½ scoops chocolate protein powder

1 banana

¼ cup shredded unsweetened coconut

2 tablespoons flaxmeal

4 ice cubes

*Add water and blend to desired consistency.

Meal 5

6 ounces salmon filet

10 stalks steamed asparagus with fresh cracked pepper and lemon

Meal 6

1 cup cottage cheese

½ cup raspberries

2 tablespoons chopped walnuts

Make meal plans using food choices like the one shown in the samples (or found at the end of the chapter) for 3 weeks. Remember to plan out all your meals for a full week in advance. If you are building muscle, continue with that plan. However, if you are not gaining muscle or are doing so at too slow a rate, you can make some simple changes to boost your calories and muscle-building capabilities.

1. Increase the size of your first solid meal following your workout. This can be done by doubling the starch portion of that meal. If you are normally eating 1 cup of rice, eat 2. If you are eating a medium-size yam, eat a large yam. In addition to doubling the starch portion, you will also want to increase your protein portion.

2. Increase the size of your breakfast. Again, as with the post-workout meal, you can double your starch and increase your protein portions of breakfast.

3. Add an extra meal. Adding an extra meal during the first 3 to 4 hours following your workout is a great way to increase your caloric consumption and fuel your body's recovery. Following one of the workout day meal plans outlined above, you could insert a grilled chicken or roasted turkey breast sandwich with spinach and tomatoes on whole-grain bread with a piece of fruit on the side. This meal would be extremely portable and easy to consume 45 to 60 minutes following your workout shake.

4. On nonworkout days, have starches during your first two meals. Having starchy carbohydrates during your first two meals will allow you to eat more carbohydrates (and calories) on your workout days to keep your body in a caloric surplus.

Here are more food options for you to build your meal plans with:

Fruits and Vegetables

Apples

Blueberries

Cantaloupe

Grapefruit

Kiwifruit

Nectarines

Oranges

Peaches

Pears

Plums

Strawberries

Watermelon

Asparagus

Beans, black (canned)

Beans, green

Broccoli

Brussels sprouts

Cabbage

Carrots

Chickpeas

Collard greens

Cucumbers

Hummus

Lettuce, romaine

Mushrooms

Onions

Peppers, green

Salsa

Spinach

Swiss chard

Tomatoes

Yellow squash

Zucchini

Protein

Bass

Beef, ground (extra-lean)

Chicken breasts

Chicken sausage

Cod

Cottage cheese (low-fat)

Egg whites

Flank steak

Halibut

Lobster

Pork loin

Protein powder

Roughy

Salmon

Scallops

Shrimp

Swordfish

Tilapia

Top round

Tuna, canned

Tuna, fresh

Turkey, ground (extra-lean)

Turkey bacon (extra-lean)

Turkey breasts

Turkey ham

Starches

Bread, whole grain

Couscous

Dextrose/maltodextrose (consume only as part of your workout nutrition)

Gatorade (consume only as part of your workout nutrition)

Oatmeal

Pasta, whole wheat

Quinoa

Rice, brown

Rice, white

Sweet potato

Tortilla, corn

Tortilla, whole wheat flour

Remember, the best way to ensure optimal results with Power Training is to adhere to the Six Pillars of Nutrition:

1. Eat five or six times a day.

2. Limit your consumption of sugars and processed foods.

3. Eat fruits and vegetables throughout the day.

4. Drink more water and cut out calorie-containing beverages (beer, soda, and so forth).

5. Focus on consuming lean proteins throughout the day.

6. Save starch containing foods until after a workout or for breakfast.

By employing these principles to your nutritional plan along with the 90 percent rule, you will be able to drastically transform your body and your health.

For more of my favorite blender bomb recipes, go to www.NakedNutritionGuide.com/PowerTraining.

POWER TRAINING
ON THE ROAD

No gym, no equipment, *no problem*! One of the most common problems for people on a serious workout schedule is going out on the road. Whether it's a business trip or a vacation, we often find ourselves with less-than-ideal training environments. I probably travel for recreation more than most people, and I can tell you that I have had to modify the Power Training workouts more than a few times. I would like to share a few of my adventures with you and the modifications that I have had to undertake. I want to preface this chapter with one simple statement: *There is no excuse for not getting in a GREAT workout, regardless of your training environment*. If a guy living in a tiny cell at Pelican Bay prison can get his workout on, so can you.

Picture yourself arriving at your hotel, excited by the fact that it has "exercise facilities" on the premises. You walk into the "gym" to find some 5- and 10-pound dumbbells and a treadmill that can't withstand your weight. What do you do? I'll tell you what I do: Go straight into McGyver mode and enjoy the challenge of seeking equipment or facilities elsewhere. Most of my "staking out" experiences come in the form of

training runs around the area. Here's a warning, though: Seriously inquire about how safe certain areas are. I once made a wrong turn in Jamaica that resulted in a little higher-intensity run than I had planned (strangely, you can run a lot faster when people are chasing you). Anyway, I can tell you that I have never, in all my years of travel, failed to find someplace to get my training in during one of these runs.

On a trip to Hong Kong in 2005, I sadly discovered that our hotel didn't have an exercise facility whatsoever. I consequently set out on my exploratory run to find one of the largest parks in Hong Kong, one with some of the best playground equipment I had ever seen! Doing chinups and parallel dips on the monkey bars as hundreds of locals practiced tai chi as the sun came up was quite an experience. It doesn't get much better than that. I have had some of my best workouts using the playground equipment at parks, elementary schools, and even kids-club facilities at vacation resorts (before they open, of course, as I wouldn't want to scare the little ones, or the counselors, for that matter).

One of my more unusual training stories comes from a 2-week trip I took to Eastern Europe in 2003. I found myself with no transportation and no gym in sight. Well, I took one of my training runs around the area and found some playground equipment at a local park and elementary school (see, if I can find this stuff in Budapest, Hungary, you should have no problem on your trips). This, however, was not the most unusual part. I came to find that the local mall never closed. In other words, the stores were locked up but one still had access to the mall. The funny thing was that the escalators still ran 24 hours a day. This was where I found one of my favorite power/cardio workouts to date: doing sprint intervals up the escalator that was going down! Here was this big guy running through this mall, sprinting up and down the escalators. Well, this must have been an unusual sight for the locals, who enjoyed watching me outrun a number of security guards who must have thought I had stolen something. While I realize that running up the down escalators is not part of the Power Training workout, it can serve as a great explosive exercise and an effective form of interval cardio.

All in all though, the trip was a good one as I did get a chance to experience a "real" training session alongside some very talented Olympic weight-lifting team members at the Hungarian Olympic Training Center in Tata.

Okay, let's get back to power training and how you might be able to modify the exercises, yet still stay relatively close to the training template. If you're in a beach area, take advantage of the sand for lower-body resistance exercises. I actually thought of one of my "15-Minute Workouts" ("Storm the Beach," *Men's Health* magazine, July/August 2004) while trying to create a comprehensive exercise routine on a beach in Kauai, Hawaii. Beaches often have useful resources like lifeguard stations, bike racks, and benches, all of which can be used for a variety of exercises like push-ups, dips, pullups, and even barrier jumps or other plyometrics. Also, don't overlook the resistive property of water or stairs, so the ocean, a pool, or the hotel stairway can also serve as tools for your training.

I suggest doing a Google or Yahoo-style search for parks and elementary schools around the area where you will be visiting, as it most likely will have playground equipment and/or fitness trails (which usually have exercise stations throughout the course). While you might not be able to perform all of your exercises, you should be able to complete most of them using just your body weight, resulting in a stellar workout.

Here is the *Men's Health* Power Training full-body workout template and some body-weight modifications you can try. Remember, you are trying to "buy time" in your conditioning status when you're in this type of situation. Your goal is to maintain and not break your workout routine. You are not expected to make gains on your squats or bench press when you are unable to actually perform these lifts without adequate load. Lastly, even if you are unable to exactly duplicate your workouts at home, you can still employ extremely effective workouts on the road.

MOVEMENT	EXERCISES	EQUIPMENT
Explosive/Power	Squat Jump, Bench Jump, Sand Jump, Stair Jump	Stairs, sand, bench, or other barrier to jump over
Knee Dominant	Squat, Split Squat, Lunges (all), Bulgarian Split Squat, Pistol Squat, Stepup	Stairs, sand, bench, or chair
Hip Dominant	Romanian Deadlift, Good Morning, Supine Hip Extension (all can be done bilaterally or unilaterally)	Bench or chair for hip extensions
Vertical Pull	Pullup, Chinup, Side-to-Side (more unilateral)	Something to hang from, chair for assistance
Vertical Push	Inverted Pushup	Bench, chair, or something similar to place feet on
Horizontal Push	Pushup, Dip, Side-to-Side Pushup (more unilateral)	Anything to place hands or feet on to make the exercises harder or easier, railings that meet at a corner or two chairs for dips
Horizontal Pull	Inverted Pullup, Side-to-Side Inverted Pullup (more unilateral), One-Arm Pull	Apparatus to hang from
Rotational	Russian Twist, Windshield Wiper	None needed
Bridge	All of the exercises!	None needed

Don't be afraid to make an exercise more difficult by turning it into hybrid exercises. Try on these for size:

• Walking lunge and side bend—also targets your core

• Pushup and row (without the dumbbells)—also targets core

• T-pushup and hold—also targets core

• Pushup into squat jump (modified burpee)—a real killer!

• Lunge up stairs

• Squat jump in sand

• Dips at a corner railing

• Pushup with feet up on a bench

• Hip extension using a chair

POWER TRAINING
15-MINUTE WORKOUTS

One challenge that often affects my training is the unpredictability of my work schedule. This sometimes leaves me with little or no time to complete a scheduled workout. My choices at this point are (1) skip the workout entirely or (2) go to the gym for a short period (not long enough to complete my entire workout). I almost always choose the latter as I think some activity is always better than no activity. As I mention earlier in the book, I like to have one day in my training where I don't perform a traditional full-body or push-pull Power Training workout. The following workouts are often performed on these days, on cardio-style days, or when there's just not enough time to complete my scheduled workout. Another benefit to these change-up workouts is the nice way they break up monotony and also give your body a chance to regroup and rest.

I have come up with five workouts that should each take you 15 minutes to complete. Don't let the fact that these are short workouts give you the impression they will be easy. These can be very difficult, depending on your intensity. The following workouts are categorized into a push, a pull, two full-body sessions, and a full-body body-weight session.

Perform 3 sets of 8 to 10 repetitions of each of the following exercises.
Keep in mind that these are all hybrid exercises.

DUMBBELL BULGARIAN SPLIT SQUAT–PRESS

Perform a standard Bulgarian split squat (page 74) with dumbbells
at your shoulders. As you descend into the squat, simultaneously
press the dumbbells overhead. Switch legs and perform the same
number of reps with the other leg.

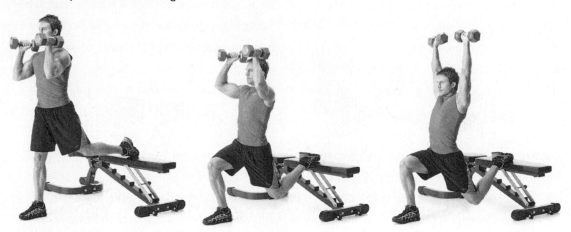

DUMBBELL SQUAT–PRESS

Stand with dumbbells resting on the front of your shoulders.
Descend into a deep squat and drive the weights overhead as you
rise from the bottom of the squat.

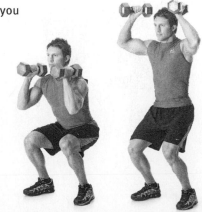

DUMBBELL ONE-ARM BENCH PRESS–ROLL ON SWISS BALL

Perform a standard one-arm bench press exercise on a Swiss ball (page 129). At the end of the press, grab the wrist of your extended arm with the opposite arm and perform a weighted roll on the ball in both directions (page 150). Perform the same number of reps with the other arm.

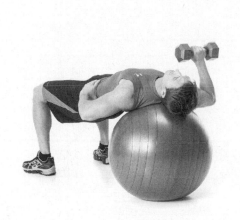
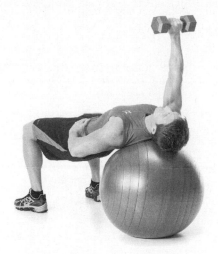
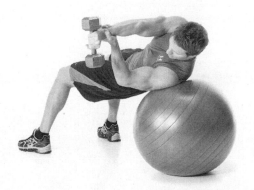
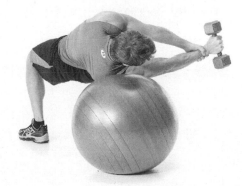

Perform 3 sets of 8 to 10 repetitions of each of the following exercises. Keep in mind all of these exercises are either complexes or hybrids.

BENT-OVER ROW + ROMANIAN DEADLIFT (COMPLEX)

Perform a standard set of bent-over dumbbell or barbell rows (page 134). At the end of the set, immediately begin your set of Romanian deadlifts (page 85).

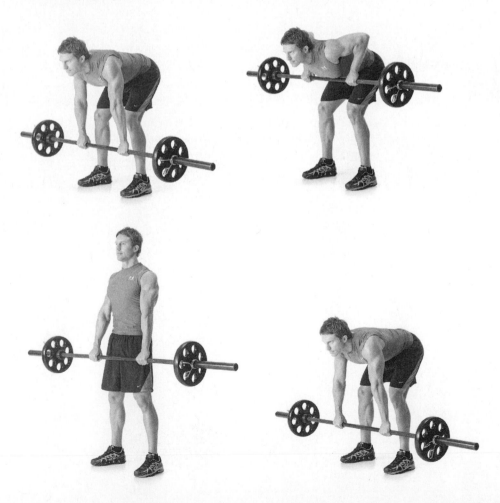

LAT PULLDOWN OR PULLUP/ CHINUP + WINDSHIELD WIPER (COMPLEX)

Perform a standard set of pulldowns or pullups/chinups (see Chapter 12). At the end of the set, immediately move to the floor and perform a set of windshield wipers (page 152).

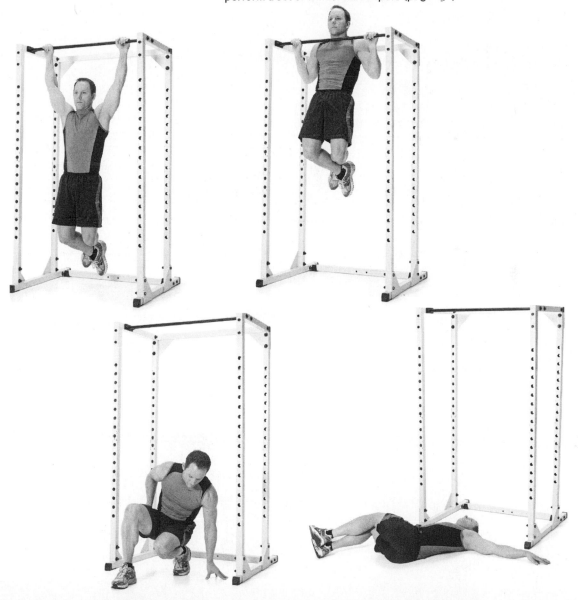

BACK EXTENSION– DUMBBELL ROW (HYBRID)

Perform a back extension (page 86) while holding a pair of dumbbells at arm's length. As you rise into the back extension, simultaneously row the dumbbells to your rib cage. Lower the dumbbells to arm's length as you lower your torso to the flexed position.

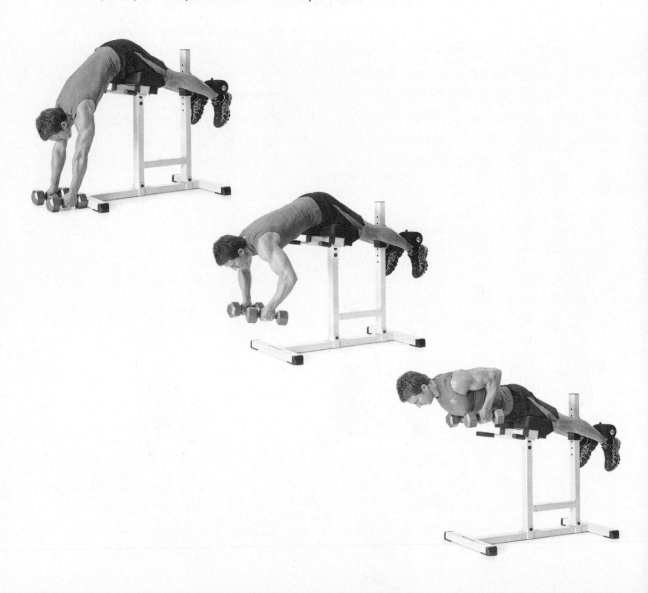

Perform 3 sets of 8 to 10 repetitions of each of the following exercises. This workout is a compilation of four hybrid exercises, and it targets just about every major muscle group.

DUMBBELL CURL–LUNGE–PRESS

Perform a biceps curl as you are stepping into a forward lunge. The dumbbells should be at your shoulders as your front foot hits the ground. From here, descend into a lunge as you simultaneously press the dumbbells overhead. Reverse the movements as you push back to the starting position. Alternate to the other leg on the next rep.

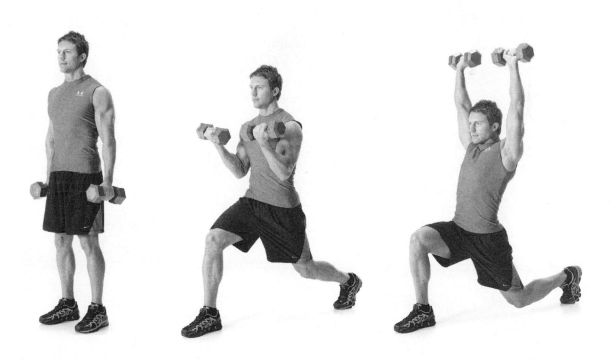

BENT-OVER ROW–BACK EXTENSION

Perform a bent-over row and while the bar is in contact with your rib cage, rise to perform a back extension (keeping the bar in contact with your body). Reverse the movements by lowering down to the bent-over position and extending your arms.

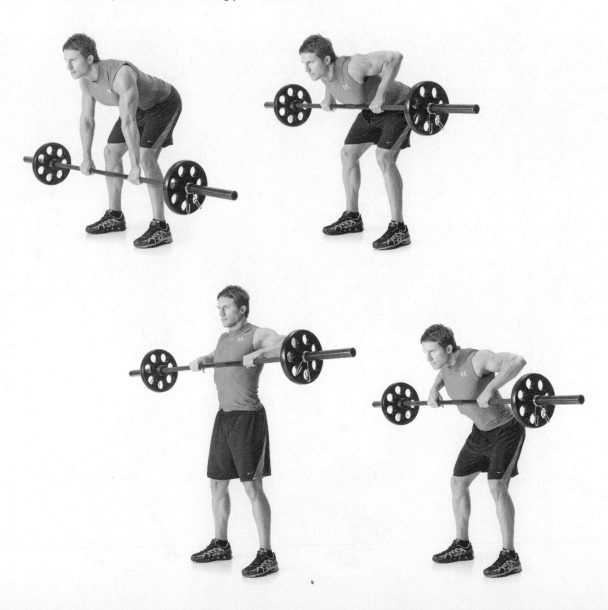

PUSHUP–CORE ROW

Place dumbells on the floor and get into a pushup position. Do a pushup and then immediately do an alternating core row.

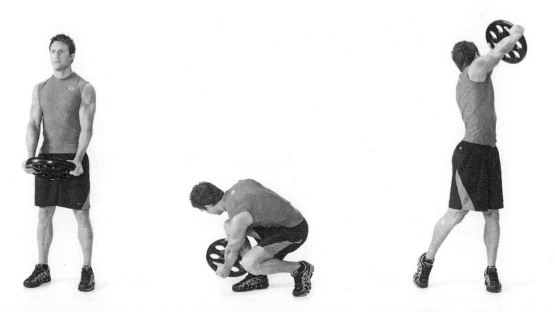

CORKSCREW

Perform a rotational corkscrew as described on page 149. Complete all prescribed reps in each direction to complete 1 set.

Perform 3 sets of 8 to 10 repetitions of each of the following exercises. These are a combination of hybrids and regular exercises that target most major muscle groups. The plyo pushup and squat jump complex should be done after completing all sets of the other exercises. They will be done for 1 set from 10 reps down to 1 rep.

CABLE SQUAT–ROW (HYBRID)

Using a cable stack machine with a bar attachment or a two-handle setup, hold the bar or handles at arms length in front of you in a standing position. Descend into a deep squat, keeping the arms extended. As you rise from the squat, row the cable handles up to your rib cage, making sure to rise and row simultaneously.

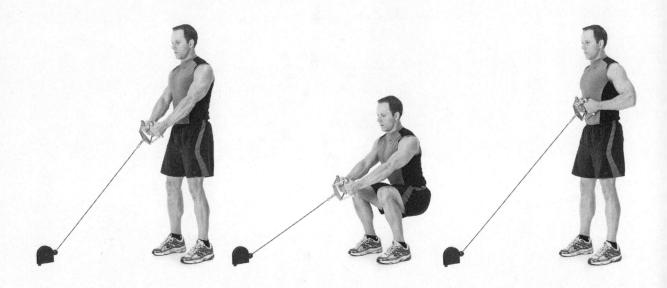

CABLE WOOD CHOP

Using a one-handle cable stack, grab the handle with both hands and perform a high-to-low style wood chop as described on page 155.

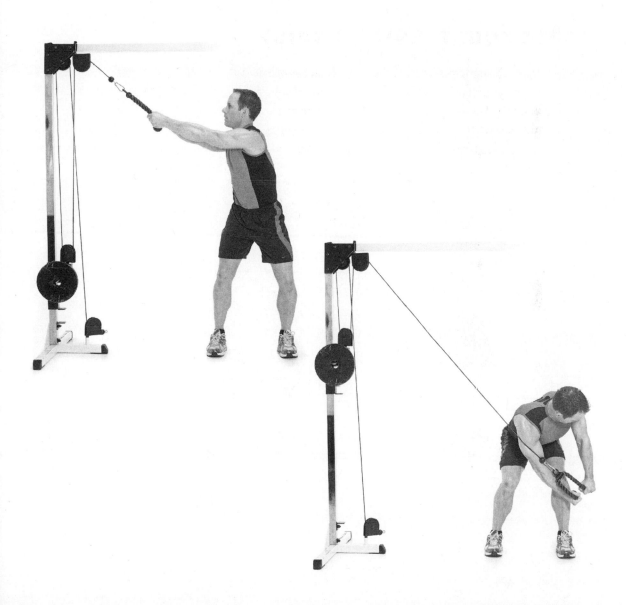

SQUAT–PRESS (HYBRID)

Using either dumbbells or a barbell from a front squat position, perform a squat and press hybrid as described on page 180.

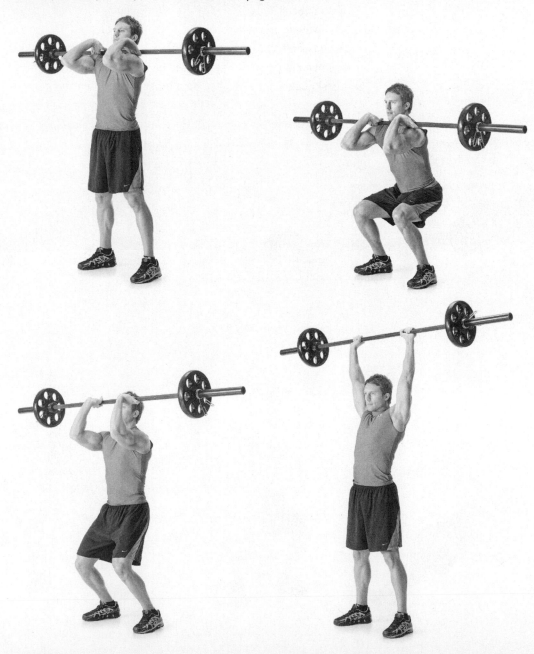

PLYOMETRIC PUSHUP
+ SQUAT JUMP COUNTDOWN

Perform 10 plyometric (clap-style) pushups, making sure to maintain a tight, rigid torso, then stand up and immediately perform 10 body-weight squat jumps with your hands on your head. Rest for 10 seconds, and then immediately go back down to the floor to perform nine plyometric push-ups followed by nine squat jumps. Continue this sequence for 8-7-6-5-4-3-2-1 repetitions. When you get to 5, eliminate the 10-second rest period and do the movements continuously. Your workout is done when you complete the countdown.

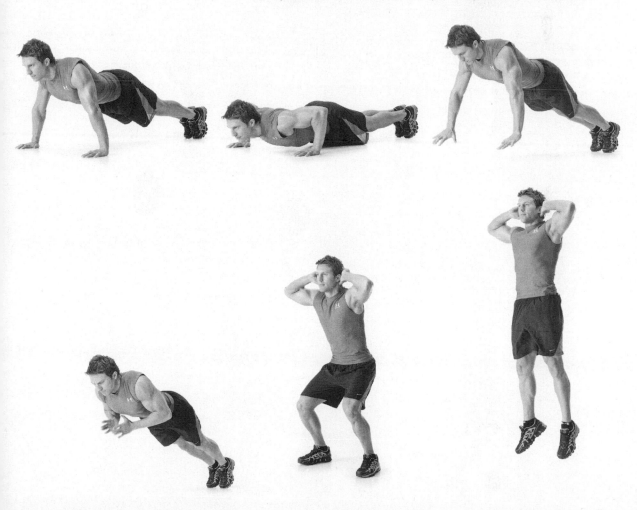

Perform 3 sets of 8 to 10 repetitions of each of the following exercises in a circuit-style fashion. Perform a set of each exercise in the order listed, back-to-back for three total circuits. Try to keep rest intervals to a minimum as there are a lot of exercises and limited time.

PULLUP OR CHINUP

Perform 8 to 10 pullups or chinups. If you can easily complete more, add weight to this exercise. See description on pages 108 and 109.

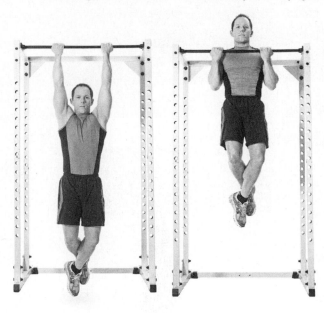

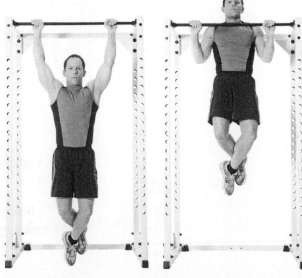

PUSHUP OR DIP

Perform 8 to 10 repetitions of either of these exercises. See descriptions in Chapter 13. If you can easily complete 8 to 10 reps, add some weight to this exercise.

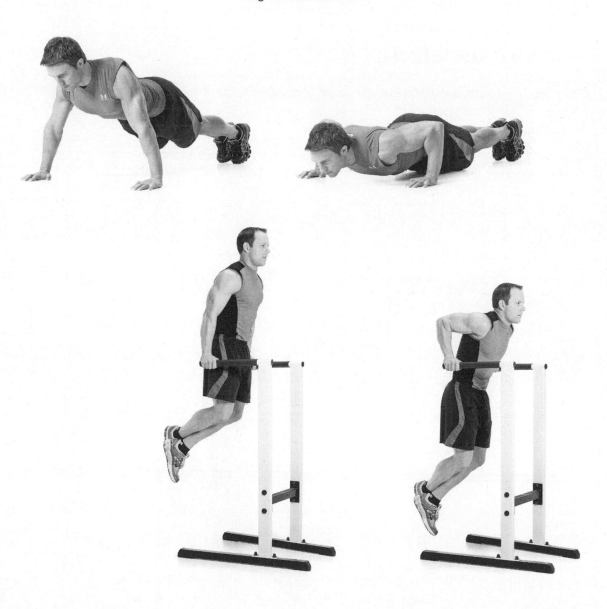

HORIZONTAL PULLUP

Perform 8 to 10 reps of this exercise as described on pages 136 and 137.

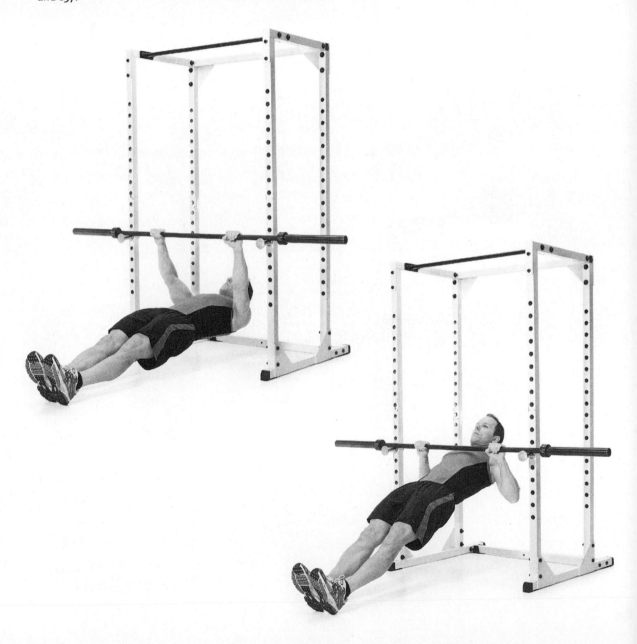

JACKKNIFE PUSHUP

Perform 8 to 10 repetitions of this exercise as described on page 101.

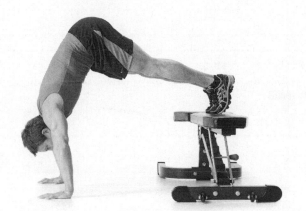
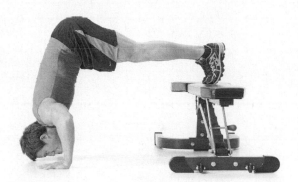

WALKING LUNGE–BEND (HYBRID)

Holding a weight above your head, perform a forward lunge. As the front foot hits the ground, you will bend in the direction of the leg that is stepping forward. Be sure to bend with shoulders square rather than rotate the torso. Reverse the movements as you step back to the starting position. Alternate to the other leg on the next rep. Keep your arms extended overhead for the entire process.

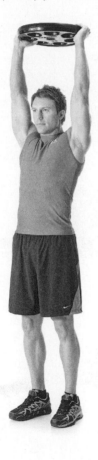
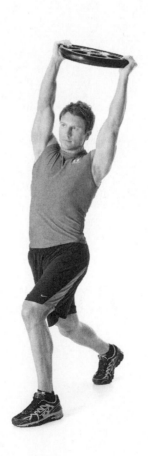
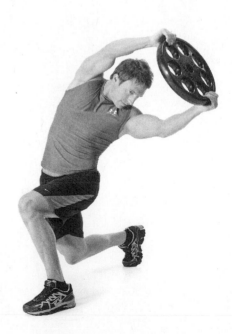

ONE-LEG GOOD MORNING OR ROMANIAN DEADLIFT

As described in Chapter 10, these two exercises are essentially the same depending on where you place the hands. With hands behind the head, the exercise is similar to a good morning while with arms hanging in front, the exercise resembles a Romanian deadlift.

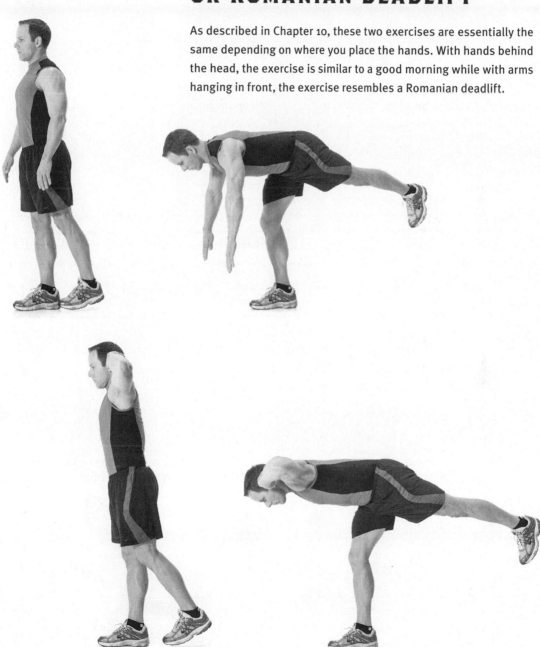

ADVANCED TRAINEE CONCEPTS—COMPLEXING EXERCISES

For advanced trainees, I have created a simple alternate option to the regular *Men's Health* Power Training workouts. This small addition will significantly increase the workload of each session to improve work capacity and power, all without significantly increasing your workout time. This option pairs an explosive exercise with a strength exercise performed back-to-back. The two exercise movements should be very similar. This training style is called *complex training* (not to be confused with the *complexes* we talked about in Chapter 17).

COMPLEX TRAINING

The concept of complex training has been around for many, many years. The idea is to pair an explosive exercise that closely resembles a strength exercise. The most common example is a squat variation and a squat jump. Another is a bench press variation and a clap, or plyometric, pushup.

While not every exercise pattern is conducive to a paired-explosive partner exercise, we can usually find something that will serve the purpose. In terms of "pairing" exercises with an explosive counterpart, I suggest complexing your explosive exercises, your vertical and horizontal pulling exercises, knee-dominant exercises, and your horizontal push exercises. In other words, you would have five complex pairs if using a full-body session (explosive, knee-dominant, vertical pull, horizontal pull, horizontal push), three complex pairs if performing a pull session (explosive, vertical pull, horizontal pull), and three complex pairs if performing a push session (explosive, knee-dominant, horizontal push). When performing these complexes, perform a set of your strength exercise, then move directly to the explosive exercise counterpart and perform a set. Rest for the prescribed time in the regular Power Training workout before beginning your next strength set. As you can see, this will add quite a bit of intensity to these exercises since we are performing an extra set of exercise without significantly adding additional rest time. I will lay out specific workout examples later in this chapter.

PLYOMETRIC PUSHUP

Perform 10 reps of this exercise as described on page 237. For less intensity than the clap-style, push off the ground without the clap. If you're looking for a more difficult exercise, try (in order of difficulty) touching your chest, touching your ears, or touching your hips at the top of the push.

MEDICINE BALL DROP

This exercise can be done with a partner or by yourself. Lie on the ground with a medicine ball on your chest. Push the ball up as high as possible, making sure to get full extension at your elbows. Catch the ball, reset, and perform the next throw. If using a partner, have the partner drop the ball as you absorb the weight of the ball and push it back up. The partner should catch the ball and drop it for the next repetition. Perform 10 repetitions.

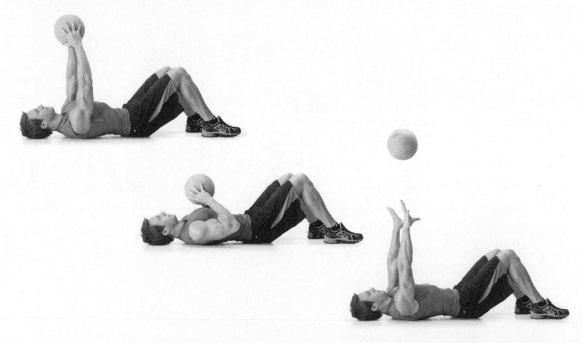

MEDICINE BALL CHEST PASS

This can be done with a partner, standing facing a wall, or by chest-passing a medicine ball down into the ground from a bent-over position. Drive the ball either into the wall or the ground as hard as possible, catching the ball on the rebound, and immediately perform another chest pass. Perform for 10 repetitions.

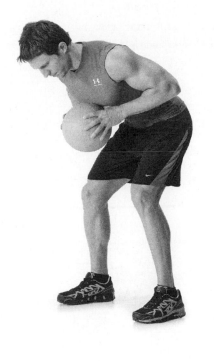
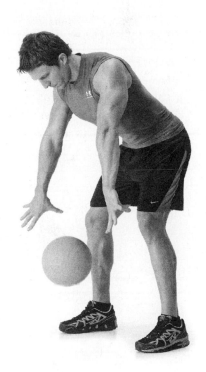

MEDICINE BALL THROW-DOWN

This is a great explosive movement that targets shoulder extension (resembling the movement of a dumbbell pullover). Stand holding a medicine ball above your head. As hard as possible, throw the ball down into the ground emphasizing the extension motion of your shoulders. With a soft ball, it will thud when it hits the ground and you can pick it up for your next rep. If using a hard rubber ball on a hard surface, the ball will bounce back up to your hands. Take advantage of the bounce and immediately move right back into the next throw-down. We will get an elastic effect if the ball bounces high enough. This way, the stretch-shortening cycle (plyometrics) will be in effect. Perform 10 repetitions.

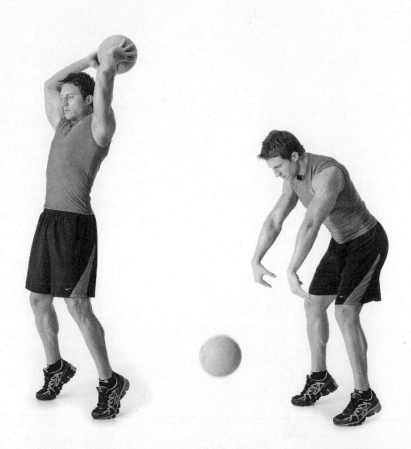

BOX OR BENCH JUMP

Set up to jump onto a bench, aerobic step, or box. Make sure the object is stable and safe before jumping. Jump as high as you can, attempting to land as lightly as possible on top of the bench or box. You should imagine that the object you are jumping on is a foot higher than it really is. Perform 5 total jumps, resetting your feet between each jump.

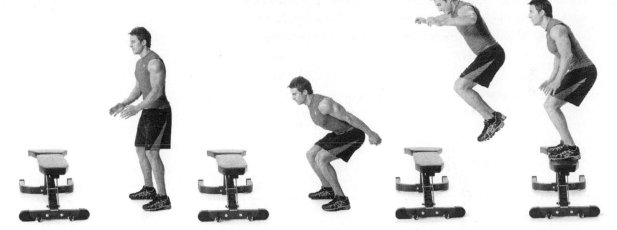

SQUAT JUMP

As described in Chapter 8, these are body-weight-only jumps with hands placed on top of your head and getting to at least a 90-degree depth before jumping up. Perform 10 jumps, making sure not to pause between jumps.

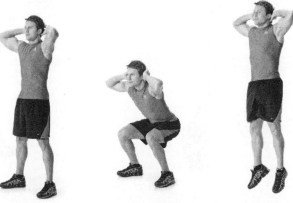

SPLIT BOX OR BENCH JUMP

Set up to jump onto a bench, aerobic step, or box. Place your left foot on top of the box and drive as hard as possible with this leg to push you up into the air. Making sure to fully extend the left knee, switch feet in the air so that you land with your right foot on the top of the box and your left foot on the floor. Absorb the jump with the leg on the box and immediately push with your right leg to perform the next jump. Perform for 10 total repetitions (5 on each leg).

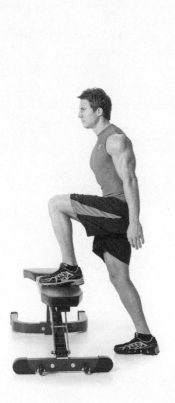
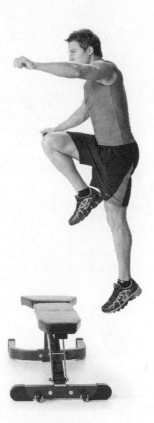
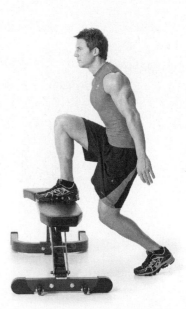

ICE-SKATER JUMP

Stand with feet close together. Push out laterally to your right, attempting to jump as far as possible. Landing on your right foot, absorb the load and immediately push back to the left, landing on your left foot. Keep this uninterrupted jumping pattern for 10 total repetitions (5 on each leg).

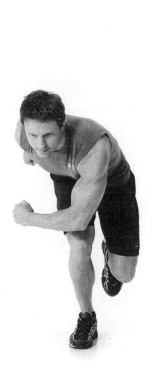
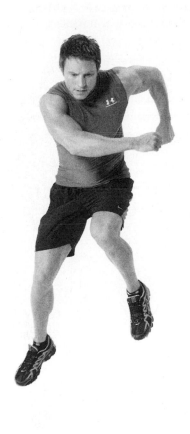
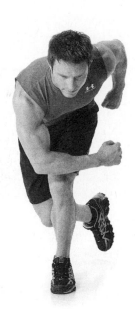

Choose from any of the explosive jumping exercises described earlier or a medicine ball scoop.

MEDICINE BALL SCOOP

If you have access to an outdoor area, this is a great explosive exercise that allows you to unload an almost identical movement as the Olympic-style exercises. With your back toward a high wall or in a completely open space, hold a medicine ball at arm's length, hanging in front of you. Squat down and lean forward. As explosively as possible, extend upward (quadruple extension), and throw (in a scooping motion) the med ball up and slightly over your head (behind), emphasizing the height of the throw. Do not attempt to catch the ball; rather, let it hit the ground and set up for the next throw. Perform 5 total "scoops."

ROMANIAN DEADLIFT JUMP SHRUG

This is very similar to the Romanian deadlift described on page 85. Using dumbbells, lower into a good Romanian deadlift and forcefully explode upward into a jump. Land and reset your body for the next rep. The objective here is to jump as high as possible with very little knee bend.

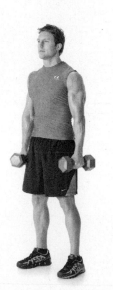
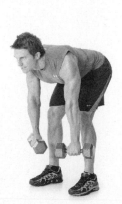
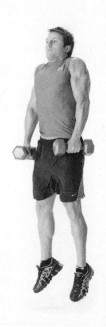

COMPLEX PAIRED EXPLOSIVE EXERCISES

We want to try to use similar movement patterns when choosing appropriate explosive exercises to pair with our strength exercises. With this in mind, these are my recommendations of explosive exercises for the power, vertical and horizontal pull, and horizontal push category exercises.

The best type of medicine ball for these explosive exercises is one made of hard rubber, as it will have a more lively bounce. We can, however, still perform explosive, uninhibited throws, and so forth, with soft medicine balls.

EXERCISE CATEGORY	SPECIFIC EXERCISES	EXPLOSIVE PAIRED EXERCISES
Horizontal Push	All menu exercises	Plyometric Pushup Medicine Ball Drop Medicine Ball Chest Pass
Horizontal Pull	All menu exercises	Medicine Ball Throw-Down
Vertical Pull	All menu exercises	Medicine Ball Throw-Down
Knee Dominant	Bilateral	Box Jump Squat Jump
Knee Dominant	Unilateral	Split Box Jump Split Squat Jump
Knee Dominant	Side Squat Side Lunge Drop Lunge Lateral Stepup	Ice Skater Jump
Explosive	All menu exercises	All explosive jumping exercises already mentioned Medicine Ball Scoop

EXAMPLE FULL-BODY SESSION WITH COMPLEXES
WORKOUT B

EXERCISE	REST	COMPLEX EXERCISE	REST
Clean Pull × 5	20–30 sec	Box Jump × 5	90 sec–2 min
Drop Lunge × 8	20–30 sec	Ice Skater Jump × 10	*1 min
Good Morning × 8	N/A	N/A	*1 min
Dumbbell Incline Bench Press × 8	20–30 sec	Plyo Pushup × 10	*1 min
Seated Row to Neck × 8	20–30 sec	Medicine Ball Throw-Down × 10	*1 min
Dumbbell Push Press × 8	N/A	N/A	*1 min
Chinup × 8	20–30 sec	Medicine Ball Throw-Down × 10	*1 min
Corkscrew × 10	N/A	N/A	*1 min
Dynamic Bridge × 30 sec	N/A	N/A	*1 min

* For 1- to 6-repetition sets, the rest period is 90 sec to 2 min.

NOTE: For those complexing a 3-day-per-week, full-body program, I suggest complexing every other week to avoid possible overtraining issues. Skip complexing sessions whenever you physically feel the need (unload).

EXAMPLE PUSH SESSION WITH COMPLEXES
WORKOUT A1

EXERCISE	REST	COMPLEX EXERCISE	REST
Hang Clean × 5	20–30 sec	Box Jump × 5	90 sec–2 min
Front Squat × 8	20–30 sec	Squat Jump × 10	*1 min
Dumbbell One-Arm Bench Press × 8	20–30 sec	Plyo Pushup × 10	*1 min
Push Jerk × 8	N/A	N/A	*1 min
Cable Wood Chop × 10	N/A	N/A	*1 min
Side Bridge + Reach × 30 sec	N/A	N/A	*1 min

* For 1- to 6-repetition sets, the rest period is 90 sec to 2 min.

EXAMPLE PULL SESSION WITH COMPLEXES
WORKOUT B2

EXERCISE	REST	COMPLEX EXERCISE	REST
High Pull × 5	20–30 sec	Squat Jump × 10	90 sec–2 min
Back Extension × 8	N/A	N/A	*1 min
Dumbbell One-Arm Row × 8	20–30 sec	Medicine Ball Throw-Down × 10	*1 min
Lat Pulldown × 8	20–30 sec	Medicine Ball Throw-Down × 10	*1 min
Swiss Ball Roll × 10	N/A	N/A	*1 min
Barbell Rollout × 60 sec	N/A	N/A	*1 min

* For 1- to 6-repetition sets, the rest period is 90 sec to 2 min.

POWER TRAINING FAQS

Q *How important are the explosive exercises that are included in this program? I don't know if I will be able to learn the Olympic lifts correctly, and I am worried that I might get hurt.*

A As I mentioned in the functional training chapter (Chapter 2), I feel that the explosive exercises are pretty important to overall fitness (so much so that I do some form of them every single training session). If you are not able to learn the technical lifts correctly (i.e., after someone has coached and observed you), stick with the pull variations, as these are very similar to traditional deadlifts with the extra-added explosive component.

Q *I notice that you talk about how unstable tools such as Swiss balls can often compromise rate of force development and the amount of load that you are able to lift. Why then would you have the Swiss ball as an option for a bench press variation exercise?*

A I do talk about how one of my pet peeves is a training program that often emphasizes instability at the cost of strength development. The Swiss ball, however, is an unstable device that actually shouldn't affect your load that significantly. The ball itself often acts as a support on the upper arms and can lead to more stability when performing dumbbell variations. Granted, if you do not have the core strength to stabilize the torso during the movement, the upper arm support is probably a moot point.

Q *The combination lifts that you talk about in the cardio section really intrigue me. Is there any way to incorporate them directly into my Power Training full-body workouts?*

A Sure, combinations like the "pure combos" are better suited for strength than complexes or hybrids, due to the load that you are able to use. Remember that variety is one of the main principles of the Power Training workouts, so feel free to use your imagination when choosing your exercises. Using combo lifts is also a great tool to keep active during unloading sessions or weeks.

Q *Is warming up really necessary? I have been training for years and have never had any injury issues associated with my muscles "not being ready."*

A In the traditional sense (i.e., 5 to 10 minutes of cardio), I think that the warmup may be a bit overrated. The problem is that everyone's body is different and some folks might feel the need to do more warming up than others. I think that the bar warmup complex plus the mobility exercises that I describe in the warmup chapter (Chapter 5) are more than sufficient to prepare the muscles for training. Just remember to perform a set or two of each particular exercise prior to your target sets (especially if you are using higher loads).

Q *I would love to be able to squat as deep as described in the Power Training squat exercises but I just can't. My heels always seem to rise as I get below parallel. Any advice?*

A A couple of recommendations here. First, try to play with the width of your base and even try to change the angle of your foot placement. If this still doesn't seem to remedy the heels coming off the floor, try placing a small weight (like a 2½-pound or at most a 5-pound) plate under your heel. Keep in mind that this is not a permanent solution; you want to develop the flexibility in your ankles, knees, and hips to improve the range of motion of your squats.

Q *I noticed that you categorized deadlifts as a knee-dominant exercise. I have always been told that they are more hip dominant. I'm confused!*

A This one has always baffled me as well. Why on earth would some training programs classify a squat as a knee-dominant movement, yet classify a traditional deadlift as a hip-dominant movement? They are almost identical movements, right? Both are driven by a forceful extension of the knee to move the weight.

Q *I am following the Power Training program to a T right now, making sure to complete all my reps and shooting to go as heavy as possible on all prescribed sets. I am getting really sore compared to how I have felt with my other training programs. Any particular reason?*

A Yes, this program is pretty tough! I mentioned earlier in this book that you will encounter discomfort pretty regularly while doing this program. Remember the overload principle and the emphasis on variation? Well, I tend to really focus on these as I see them as the keys to muscle growth and strength gains. Just keep hammering away—your body will adapt and overcome. Also, don't forget my suggestions to unload at least every 6 weeks or so.

Q *I know that you are against isolated exercises, but is it bad if I do some biceps curls at the end of my pull workouts?*

A There is a place for just about everything. I am 100 percent fine with one doing additional isolated work if one feels the need. From a functional point of view, I don't see much merit in it, and time tends to be a factor in most people's training schedules. Remember, however, that I did talk about how isolation exercises can bring added hypertrophy (i.e., bodybuilders). As long as it doesn't interfere with your main workout, knock yourself out.

Q The menu lists for most of the Power Training categories are pretty long. I know that you recommend trying all or most of the exercises throughout your training cycles, but what if I really love only one or two of the exercises on the lists?

A I understand that human nature will drive us toward familiarity and comfort zones. The menu in the Power Training is there to give you lots of freedom to choose. It is also your choice of whether you want to do certain exercises. I would still recommend that you try most of them along the way, but if you are a creature of habit and you're still feeling challenged with your choices, then stay the course.

Q I am on a 4-day push-pull workout split (Monday, Tuesday, Thursday, Friday). If I miss, say, Tuesday's workout, should I just come back on Wednesday to complete it and then take Thursday off or should I just wait until Thursday and do Thursday's scheduled workout?

A Good question. You can just complete it the next day (Wednesday) and then get right back on schedule and do the scheduled workout on the very next day. Your other option is to complete your missed workout the next day and then push Thursday and Friday's workouts to Friday and Saturday. I personally would prefer to get back on schedule by training consecutively on Wednesday, Thursday, and Friday.

Q My workouts seem to be taking longer than the estimated times listed in this program. What am I doing wrong?

A Most likely you are resting too long between sets (which is common). Try timing your rest intervals and keeping a pretty tight schedule. You should save some time by doing this.

Q I have read in other books and magazines that doing 3 sets of 10 and 10 sets of 3, with similar loads, are the same thing since the total volume and workload is the same. Is it okay for me to do this with the Power Training exercises?

A Nonsense. You'd be spinning your wheels by doing sets of 3 with your 10-repetition maximum. You would be getting nothing out of this type of training regardless of how hard you were to push the light load. You'd be totally ignoring the overload principle, which if you remember is the number-one principle for building strength, with this type of training. Furthermore, you could actually do 10 sets of 3 repetitions with close to your 3RM and get strength benefits, but remember that muscular strength and muscular hypertrophy are attained through totally different training methods.

Q I train at home and I don't have a squat rack. Any advice on how I can still do heavy squats?

A This could be a problem. Without racks, you will have to lift the load to your shoulders, and for most of us, this is difficult as we are able to squat much more than we can lift off the ground and place on our shoulders. Try sticking to the single-leg movements for your heavier loads. You can also do heavy clean-grip deadlifts (just be sure to emphasize the knee extension and not turn it into a Romanian deadlift).

Q I have been sick for more than a week and have been unable to train at all. I have missed an entire week's worth of Power Training workouts. Have all my gains now been compromised?

A Being sick is a part of life. Quite often we miss valuable training sessions due to illness or other reasons. Your main concern should be to get healthy and get back in the gym when your body is ready. No sense in trying to train when your body is in a funk and unable to handle the exercise.

Q I have always trained using very slow tempos (3 to 4 seconds eccentric and 3 to 4 seconds concentric). In the Power Training program, you tell us that it should take approximately 2 seconds to complete a repetition. Can I expect the same results if I stay with my slower tempos?

A No. While deliberately slow concentric and eccentric muscular movements may result in quicker fatigue and compromised loads, they don't result in greater strength or size gains. Our goal in Men's Health Power Training is to train with as much load as our bodies can handle. We also want to try to move through concentric phases with as much force as possible; this is not possible if we are deliberately moving slow. Many believe that training at slow paces leads to more effective workouts due to the perceived exertion at the end of sets. This is not true. Very light loads can lead to dramatic fatigue if we move slow enough. This, however, doesn't mean that is a better training method.

Q I understand the Power Training philosophy on machines and how you recommend unsupported training whenever possible. Some days I am just lazy and my gym has some of the most movement-specific machines around. Is it okay to occasionally do my Power Training workout using mostly these machines?

A Hey, you're human! I have been in that situation many, many times. While the gold standard will always be free-weight, unsupported exercises, who's to say that we can't dabble in some of those fancy machines once in a while? Have fun but don't get too comfy on that cushy vertical chest press!

Q Is training unilaterally really that important for my progress?

A I really think so. The effects are quite different on the central nervous system and on the muscles as well. As I mention in the book, unilateral training allows us to see imbalances and forces our limbs to function independently (which is a big change for most people). Keep alternating between bilateral and unilateral and I guarantee you will see great results at the end of each training cycle.

Q My goal is to get as big as possible. I am not interested in training for performance or function. Is the Power Training program going to help me reach my goals?

A Probably not. In the functional training chapter (Chapter 2), I emphasize the philosophy of this program; cosmetic, mannequin-style muscles are not at all important to me. While I know that those on this program will see great physique changes (as athletes do with this training program), those whose goals are associated with maximum hypertrophy and little to no functional real-life strength will probably find better results in a traditional high-intensity training program.

Q I notice that you don't have crunches or situps on the Power Training menu. Are they bad for you? What if I do some additional crunches at the end of my workouts?

A No, crunches are not bad for you. When laying out my program, I made decisions based on function, effectiveness, and time. While crunches can build specific strength to that movement and can result in hypertrophy in muscles associated with trunk flexion, I felt that they were not an essential part of this program. As with isolation work, I am not at all against people doing additional crunch work at the end of training sessions.

Q I am having a difficulty differentiating between the split squat and the forward and reverse lunge.

A Common question. While they may look very similar, they are very different exercises. A lunge by nature needs to involve an actual lunging motion (either forward, backward, or lateral). In other words, you are going somewhere with one leg and pushing back to the starting position. With a split squat, your feet are fixed and the body is moving directly up and down. In addition, you are also attempting to push with both legs simultaneously. This is why one is a unilateral and the other is a bilateral exercise.

Q In the advanced Power Training program you talk about complexing weight exercises with explosive exercises. You recommend short rest periods between strength and explosive exercises. Will I get more out of this training if I cut out the rest periods completely?

A The recommendation for this short 20- to 30-second rest period after the paired strength exercise is to give your body a little time to recover as you set up for the explosive exercise. Otherwise, your explosive sets tend to get sloppy. Remember to rest for the full length of time prescribed after the explosive exercise (before your next strength set).

Q You mention unloading at 6 or 12 weeks of training. Do I really have to unload if I feel fine?

A Due to the constant variations and the emphasis to push the loads during workouts, there is a pretty slim chance that you will find yourself feeling refreshed or pretty good after completing 12 weeks of Power Training workouts. Even if this is the case, I would still suggest unloading for at least a week to let the body recover a bit. As I mentioned in the program design chapter, rest is a good thing and we can often make bigger gains if we take advantage of the restoration process. This is why I suggest unloading about every 6 weeks or so.

Q *What's so different between your alternating linear periodization and traditional undulating periodization?*

A Traditional undulating periodization changes training emphasis either weekly or even as frequently as workout to workout. As I mentioned in the program design chapter (Chapter 4), I do not believe that this gives us enough time to adjust to specific loads, and it can lead to less than optimal results. With the alternating linear periodization that I use in the Power Training program, we still fluctuate our loads and volumes, only we do it at 3-week intervals, thus allowing adequate time for our bodies to adjust, adapt, and improve before moving to the next phase.

Q *I use a 3-day-per-week, full-body program and want to start complexing some of my exercises to add intensity to my training sessions. Will this be too much work? Am I setting myself up for overtraining problems?*

A While everyone's body is different, I suggest complexing every other week when using a full-body, 3-day program. This is just to make sure that we err on the side of caution. Another suggestion is to complex train every other workout. In either case, you would be getting three complex sessions every 2 weeks.

Q *What are your suggestions for cardio training in conjunction with the Power Training program?*

A Well, this really depends on your goals. If you are trying to reduce body fat, I suggest adding 12 to 15 minutes of high-intensity, interval-style cardio at the end of each training session. I will also suggest designating at least 1 day per week when you are not performing the Power Training workouts to focus on cardio (using these training methods). If you are trying to bulk, I would not do much cardio at all.

Q *Any suggestions for adding some volume to my hypertrophy phases?*

A I believe that the volume in the program will be sufficient, but you can perform sort of a "giant set" (back-to-back sets targeting the same muscle movement) with your exercises if you feel the need to add some volume. Make any extra exercises body-weight variations. Try a pushup set paired with your horizontal push, a body-weight set of chinups between your sets of lat pulldowns, or even a body-weight lunge between sets of squats. Simply performing sets of 5 to 10 reps with these basic exercises will add significant volume to your training. Move directly to the body-weight exercise after your regular exercise (without rest) and rest for the prescribed time after the body-weight exercise before your next regular set.

INDEX

Underscored page references indicate boxed text and tables. **Boldface** references indicate illustrations.